Healthcare of the Well Pet

Healthcare of the Well Pet

Caroline Jevring
BVetMed, MRCVS

Thomas E. Catanzaro
DVM, MHA, FACHE
Diplomate, American College of Healthcare Executives

 W. B. SAUNDERS COMPANY LTD
London • Edinburgh • New York • Philadelphia • Sydney • Toronto

W.B. SAUNDERS An imprint of Harcourt Brace and Company Limited

© Harcourt Brace and Company 1999

Ⓡ is a registered trademark of Harcourt Brace and Company Limited

The right of Caroline Jevring and Thomas E. Catanzaro to be identified as authors of this work has been asserted by them in accordance with the Copyright, Design and Patents Act 1988

Firsty published 1999

ISBN 0-7020-23930

The image used on the cover of this product was modified using original images from MasterPhotos ANML0049 JPG. MasterPhotos is a copyrighted and a registered trademark of IMSI, 75 Rowland Way, Novato, CA 94945 USA.

British Library Cataloguing in Publication Data
A catalogue record for this book is available from the British Library

Library of Congress Cataloging in Publication Data
A catalog record for this book is available from the Library of Congress

Note
Medical knowledge is constantly changing. As new information becomes available, changes in treatment, procedures, equipment and the use of drugs become necessary. The editors/authors/contributors and the publishers have, as far as it is possible, taken care to ensure that the information given in the text is accurate and up to date. However, readers are strongly advised to confirm that the information, especially with regard to drug usage, complies with latest legislation and standards of practice.

The publisher's policy is to use paper manufactured from sustainable forests

Typeset by IMH(Cartrif), Loanhead, Scotland
Printed in China

Contents

Preface

Pets have moved from the backyard into the bedroom
Marty Becker, DVM

That veterinarians should promote healthcare for pets is obvious – or is it?

Apparently not. Veterinarians are not taught about healthcare at University, nor about how to educate clients through excellence in communication, nor even about the value of pets to human health (the basis of farm animal healthcare and food production programmes). Most importantly of all, veterinarians still do not fully appreciate the importance of the family-pet bond – a relationship in which the veterinarian plays a vital, integral and exciting role.

Of course, veterinarians *have* practised pet healthcare to some extent over the last few decades. A recent visit to rural Thailand clearly showed the difference between the prematurely aged, mangy, worm-ridden village dogs and cats which roam their streets, compared to the sleek, healthy, vaccinated, parasite-free pets which walk on ours. The problem is, today's veterinarians tend to stop at the 'routine stuff' such as vaccinations and parasite control recommendations, whereas they – or, better, their staff – could *actively* help owners to prevent dental disease; prevent behaviour problems through pet selection and appropriate management; prevent unwanted pregnancies and sex-hormone related diseases such as pyometra; and reduce the incidence of obesity, FLUTD, and growth problems through optimal diet. They could make accurate recommendations about exercise, grooming, and the management of the pet's micro-environment. They could *actively* work with pet owners to help them both enhance their pets' health, and enjoy a richer more rewarding relationship with their pet.

What's stopping them? Perhaps it's a feeling that healthcare won't work – after all, look at the lack of success of human healthcare programmes, or that owners aren't interested, or that it isn't the job for which veterinarians have been trained. However, owners really *do* care about their pets – statistics prove an ever-increasing number regard their pets as family members, and veterinarians really *are* the animal healthcare experts – there is no other profession or training that gives the same in depth and comprehensive understanding of husbandry, disease prevention and health management.

I suspect the real reason is that veterinarians are not sure *how* to actively practice healthcare. This book aims to fill the gaps that arise during a conventional veterinary training, and to inspire veterinarians and their staff to work more effectively with owners on wellness healthcare for their pets. The contributory authors, all world experts in their fields, are bound by a common passion – that health and well-being is the right of every animal, that a rich and rewarding relationship is the right of every pet owner, and that the person most able to enrich this miraculous bond is the veterinarian. I hope you find it stirs this passion within you, too.

Caroline Jevring, BVetMed, MRCVS
January, 1999

When Caroline Jevring asked me to co-author this text for release in Europe, we discussed 'Preventive Medicine and Wellness Healthcare Needs' as the theme. I had built and opened veterinary hospitals in the Rheinpfalz of Germany from 1985 to 1989, and knew there was an evolution from curative care to wellnesss care coming to Europe. The United States had undergone this wellness healthcare evolution since I returned from Germany, and I considered it an honour to be asked to share in the developement of this text.

I have had four design, leadership and management texts published in the last two years and four more are in production, but this text is a cornerstone of every veterinary practice as we enter the new millenium. Currently, about 80% of the pets accessing veterinary care are being brought in by clients who want them to stay healthy. These pets have family-member status and deserve the professional care to maintain a good quality of life. The clients deserve the peace of mind associated with keeping their pets healthy. The veterinary practice deserves the satisfaction of well pet care, including charging an equitable fee for their professional support of this quest.

This text introduces the concept of wellness healthcare delivery. We include details of dental conditions and levels of hospitalization (differential pricing is then possible). We discuss the aging pet, as well as puppy and kitten programs (the traditional wellness programs). All animals must eat, so nutritional counselling is a wellness need, as is reproduction and behaviour management efforts. If we look at the evolution of human healthcare, friends, we can see what type of companion animals deserve. It is our hope that this text awakens the European and international veterinary community, showing that curative medicine (fees by the hundred-weight value) should give way to the subjective value of wellness healthcare delivery (at a fair value) to the companion animal.

Thomas E. Catanzaro, DVM, MHA, FACHE
Diplomate, American College of Healthcare Executives
January, 1999

Acknowledgements

Two decades ago Dr Leo Bustand started the Delta Society, an international clearing house for information about human–animal interaction in the environment. Early in this Century Dr Albert Schweitzer (1875-1965) wrote of the origin of 'Reverence for Life', which is the basis for his most important book, The Philosophy of Civilization. The following excerpts are from this report (1915), which are more relevant today than when this article was originally written by Dr Schweitzer.

> From childhood, I felt a compassion for animals. Even before I started school, I found it impossible to understand why, in my evening prayers, I should pray only for human beings. Consequently, after my mother had prayed with me and had given me a good-night kiss, I secretly recited another prayer, one I had composed myself. It went like this: 'Dear God, protect and bless all living beings. Keep them from evil and let them sleep in peace'.
>
> The founding societies to protect animals, which was actively promoted during my youth, made a great impression on me. People actually dared to announce publicly that compassion toward animals was a natural thing, a sign of true humanity and that one must not hide one's feelings about it. I believed that a light was beginning to shine in the darkness of ideas, and that it would glow with ever greater brilliance.

The Scouting movement, founded by Lord Baden-Powell in England in the first decade of this Century, has one point of the Scout Law reinforcing the kindness to animals as a core value for every day in the Scouting movement.

There is a long history of concern for animal welfare and now that is being converted to wellness healthcare by the patient advocates of the veterinary profession. To each veterinarian who accepts this evolutionary and revolutionary role, we thank you.

Caroline and Tom Cat

List of Contributors

Caroline Jevring
Skyttevahen 9 A
Nordic Connection AB
133 36 Saltsjobaden
Sweden

Thomas E. Catanzaro
1217 Washington Avenue
Golden
Colorado 80401-1144
USA

Dr Ceciha Gorrell
17 Burnt House Lane
Pilley
Nr Lymington
Hants
SO41 5QN
UK

Sarah Heath BVSc MRCVS
Behaviour Referrals
11 Cotebrook Drive
Upton
Chester
Cheshire
CH2 1RA
UK

Dr David Lloyd
Dept. Small Animal Medicine &
    Surgery
Royal Veterinary College
Hawkshead Lane
North Mymms
Hatfield
Hertfordshire
AL9 7TA
UK

Why Healthcare for the Well Pet?

Caroline Jevring, Thomas E. Catanzaro

What really raises one's indignation against suffering is not suffering intrinsically, but the senselessness of suffering.
Nietzsche

Where the knowledge and skills exist to prevent illness, disease and suffering, it is negligent not to use them. Veterinarians daily see pets that are suffering. Obesity and nutritional inadequacies, dental disease, poor parasite control, breed-related physical problems, behavioural disorders and so on are not true diseases – they are a lack of wellness or health. Veterinarians have the *knowledge and skills* to prevent this suffering, they have the necessary *ability and training* – and they also have the *responsibility* to care for animals. Both ethically and morally all veterinary effort should be directed towards preventing disease and suffering, and promoting health in animals: to promote what is *best* for the pet.

So, why aren't veterinarians doing it?

The image still fostered by the profession is that veterinary clinics are places to bring sick animals for treating. But we will soon be in the twenty-first century – this image harks back to the nineteenth!

Is wellness care in companion animal practice really such a radical concept?

No! Disease prevention and health management has long been the focus of veterinary care in farm animal practice. Economic pressures were the greatest influence on changing veterinary attitudes in this situation. Some of the pressures for change in the world of the companion animal veterinarian are illustrated in Fig. 1.1.

It is no longer appropriate for veterinarians simply to fix sick pets. A pet is, more often than not, a member of the family. Owners want to help their pets to have a good quality of life, and the knowledge exists to help them do so. Owners want pet healthcare.

I

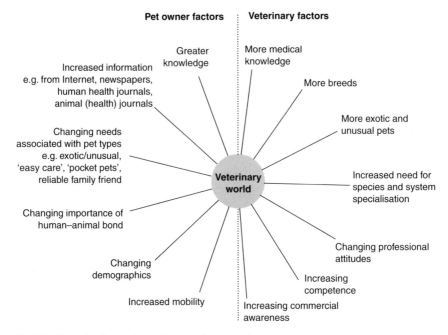

Fig. 1.1 Some key factors influencing veterinary practice.

In human medicine in the United States, *healthcare*, as one word, means a total medical, psychological and physical wellness mission. In food animal medicine, 'preventive healthcare' is the basis for comprehensive and integrated herd health programmes seen as 'dollars per kilo' profit by producers. In companion animal practices 'preventive care' once meant a strong vaccination or worming programme, but, as this book highlights, this is no longer enough.

Wellness healthcare incorporates all aspects of pet ecosystem management to help pets live longer, healthier and richer lives. Instead of dealing with each preventive healthcare issue separately, wellness healthcare combines them to give total healthcare. This is presented to pet-owners in the form of organised programmes. Owners are integral to the success of these programmes as they are essential members of the healthcare team made up of the veterinarian, the practice staff, and the owner and family.

Wellness healthcare is not an option. As a result of better protection against killer diseases through vaccination, better nutrition, and better parasite control, pets are living longer. Average life-spans have increased so that, for example, care of the older pet is a real need requiring specialist knowledge and skills for the management of age-related and geriatric diseases. The aim with senior healthcare is not 'cure', though, but management and helping the pet to lead as comfortable and full a life as possible.

The changing relationship of owners with their pets means that owners *want* their pets to live long and healthy lives. In many cases, pets are as important to them as people, and often serve as substitutes for 'family'. The veterinarian is integral to this relationship. As the only person qualified to give the correct advice about the health and welfare of animals, the veterinarian must be involved from *before* birth through the animal's whole life until *after* death, from advising on breed selection and pre-natal care of the mother through maintaining health by correct ecosystem management throughout the pet's life, to helping owners cope with the death and the grieving associated with loss of a dear friend.

Wellness healthcare requires a *proactive* approach that is very different from traditional *reactive* disease treatment. Veterinarians have in the past focused on the aspect of 'helping the sick', and so owners are not used to coming to them with healthy pets. Veterinarians need to work hard to change this view before it is too late and their leadership position is lost to people less qualified to advise accurately on animal care and welfare.

There are three reasons why promoting health rather than treating sickness is essential in companion animal practice:
- it is best for the animals;
- it is best for the owners;
- it is best for the practice.

Let's look at each of these issues in more depth.

Best for the animals

Wellness healthcare goes a long way beyond preventive healthcare in that it considers the whole of the pet's background and environment in relation to its health. The aim is to produce physically and mentally healthier pets that enjoy life and are a pleasure to own.

Many of the conditions healthcare programmes prevent or, at best, manage cause suffering and distress to the pet. Animals are adepts at hiding pain. Often this is not appreciated until the source of the pain is removed surgically or medically and their behaviour changes dramatically when owners comment that their pet has got 'a new lease of life' or behaves 'like a puppy/kitten' again. For example, a distressingly high proportion of pets suffer from neglected mouths which give constant discomfort. After appropriate treatment owners report that their pet's temperament has improved, and that it eats well again, and that 'he's back to his old self'. Many of these neglected mouths could have been prevented by actively advising owners *before* purchase about the potential problems particular breeds may expect – toy breeds generally need far more dental attention than large breeds – and then encouraging prophylactic dental home care which is regularly monitored by the practice from the day of purchase.

Another example of the powerful effects of wellness healthcare is where practices offer an advisory service for pet selection and behaviour management. In many countries the 'disposable pet' syndrome is a major problem. Pets that are mismatched with their owners are at best rehomed, at worst killed. The pet advisory service includes consideration of the owner's needs for a pet, and the time and money they could realistically spend on a pet. It also considers breed characteristics (size, coat length, temperament, etc.) and matches these to owner requirements. Prospective owners learn about normal behaviour for their new pet so that they can integrate that into their expectations. Informed and accurate advice gives the pet a better start and a better chance in life.

Best for the owners

Pets are good for people (Fig. 1.2). Interactions with pets have at least seven psychological and social functions that affect human longevity and decrease morbidity. These include:

- providing companionship;
- keeping people active;
- stimulating care-giving activity;
- making their owners feel safe;
- permitting the exchange of affectionate touch;

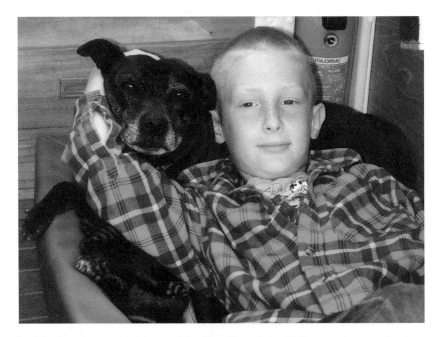

Fig. 1.2 Pets give unrestricted unconditional love. The relationship between the pet and each family member differs according to their needs: a companion, a playmate, a watchdog, and so on. To communicate effectively with the family veterinarians need to appreciate the different roles a pet can play.

- being an interesting visual object (so relieving boredom);
- being a stimulus to exercise.

Added to these is the effect of pets on health. There is both a direct and an indirect relationship between health and pet ownership, for example on the survival and recovery rates of patients with heart surgery, from stress reduction and increased exercise.

The relationship between man and animals is ancient and complex, and unusual in that it is a cross-species form of attachment. Attachment behaviour normally derives from a need to keep individuals together and acts as a mechanism for social cohesion to enhance survival. For example, people tend to be very attached to their own children. This is encouraged by the child's natural morphology and behaviour – the appealing rounded head, crying when abandoned, seeking physical contact and reassurance, and so on. Pets maintain a sort of infantile state of innocent dependence that stimulates human instincts to offer support and protection. 'Babyish' physical and mental characteristics have been selectively bred for in those species with whom humans have the most contact, especially dogs. Many toy breeds, for example, retain the domed skull shape of young animals, the short legs and small size which makes them easy to pick up and cuddle, and show dependent, clinging, 'baby' behaviour.

Pets respond to people. They appear happy when their owner comes home, sad when the owner departs, and look guilty for doing something wrong. They enthusiastically seek out and greet people, and can elicit guilt feelings through facial expression or by crying plaintively. They often like to maintain physical contact for prolonged periods of time, something that is almost impossible with most humans in our society today, and they are non-judgemental. Devoted owners anthropomorphise their pet's behaviour and impose characters on them by, for example, talking to them and making up their supposed responses. For many people, pets are members of or even substitutes for their family, in some cases to the extent that the pet can mean more to them than any living human (Fig. 1.3).

This attachment behaviour between owner and pet can persist even when the pet exhibits difficult or problem behaviour. It depends on factors such as how close the owner's involvement is with important others (people or animals), and the functions of the pet. Transactions between humans and animals provide safety, intimacy, kinship and constancy.

Some of the roles of a companion animal

Pets play a different role for people at different stages of their lives. As well, to each member of a family they can be something different – a companion or another child to the mother, a source of exercise to the father, a playmate or friend to the child, a grandchild to the elderly. We believe that pets give us companionship, friendship and happiness. They also make us feel safe – especially at night and if we are alone. They

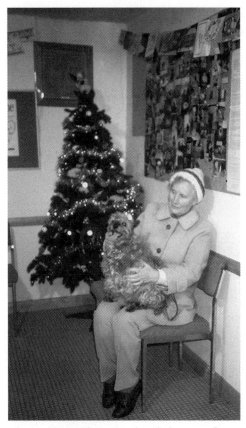

Fig. 1.3 People form close and loving lifetime bonds with their pets. Courtesy of Millhouse Veterinary Surgery, Kings Lynn.

> *make us feel important and increase our self-confidence, and sometimes, unfortunately, they relieve our hostilities by acting as our scapegoats. They also play with us, and so allow expression of the eternal child inside most adults. Above all, pets allow us to love and be loved.'*
> Salmon and Salmon, in *New Perspectives on our Lives with Companion Animals*, 1983, p. 265

The bond that exists between man and animal originated as a need for a help-mate (guard, herder, beast of burden, rodent controller) and has now evolved, in some cases, to child-replacement or only friend. At the opposite end of the spectrum, large aggressive breeds of dog may be selected to represent an extension or reflection of the aggressive side of their owner's personality, or to mask image inadequacies.

Keeping busy enhances the longevity of older people and owning a pet can serve this function. For retired people, a pet makes life more interesting and complex, and encourages the owner to maintain a daily routine. This helps to overcome feelings of uselessness and depression arising from missing the meaningful activity that came from their job.

Personal safety is a worry for many people who live in increasing isolation in an increasingly violent society. Older people in particular can feel trapped and helpless, fearing attack when alone. A companion animal, especially a dog, provides a feeling of security, and serves as a deterrent to thieves and muggers.

Pets provide companionship, someone to talk to, and someone to touch that can reduce the feeling of loneliness many people experience in modern society. Affectionate caressing releases endorphins in the brain which have a soothing and calming influence in the body, slowing heart rate and breathing rate. The vast majority of pet-owners talk to their pet and use a special language (Fig. 1.4): sentences are broken into small series of words usually phrased as a question and concluding with a rising intonation followed by a pause, as though waiting for the pet to reply.

Pets enable owners to have more social contact with other people, often other pet-owners, and have a role in helping maintain physical fitness. People also play

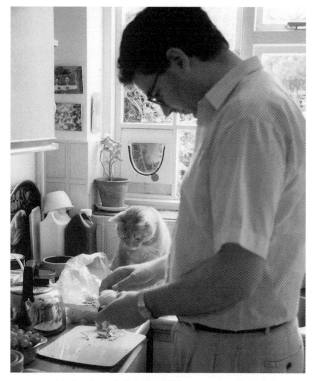

Fig. 1.4 Pets are non-critical and non-judgemental. Most owners talk to their pets as though they were people, and love giving treats. © Ann F. Stonehouse.

with their pets. Games are typically light-hearted, and accompanied by laughter, providing another chance for exercise and relaxation. But pet-owners also play passively with their pets, and the pet becomes, in effect, an extension of the person. This situation is often seen in veterinary surgeries where people sit with unfocused eyes playing with, stroking or rolling the pet's hair between their fingers. These gestures are quite similar to the displacement gestures that children and animals direct against their own person during times of tension.

Pet-facilitated therapy (PFT) is increasingly widely used in nursing homes for the elderly, helping mentally and physically disabled children and adults, and in other situations where people are institutionalised. For one specific group of patients – children with cerebral palsy and spastic muscle disorders – riding has proved to be a very effective way of improving muscle control, providing motivation and enhancing self-image.

The role of guide dogs and hearing dogs has opened up and enriched the lives of many visually and hearing impaired people. A recent two-year study in America showed that specially trained dogs helping people with disabilities in their homes not only improved the quality of the person's life significantly, but also saved about £900 per year per person in social costs. The dogs were better than paid healthcare workers because they provided their owners with increased self-esteem, well-being, community integration, and control. They helped their owners accomplish tasks and gave emotional support.

Interestingly, trainers can also benefit from contact with pets. Work done with prisoners in the United States Army showed that those selected to train therapy pets benefited enormously in developing their own social role and responsibilities when they eventually returned to society.

The role of the veterinarian in the human–animal bond

In addition to caring for animal patients, today's veterinarian is responsible, directly or indirectly, for maintaining and improving the physical, mental, and emotional well-being of his or her clients.

Appreciating the strength and complexity of the bond between people and their pets is a very important part of practising veterinary medicine. As spokesperson for the health and welfare of animals, the veterinarian is an integral part of this bond. In fact, companion animal practice is founded upon the family–pet–vet bond. By understanding how important a pet is to the owner the veterinarian is then in a position to help the animal most effectively.

Veterinarians can show their appreciation of and understanding for the human–animal bond in many ways. For example, it has been shown that direct interaction with friendly pets causes people's blood pressure to fall, their face muscles to relax, and they tend to smile more often – effects not as marked when interacting with other people. Veterinarians who take their own pets to work or have a friendly practice mascot demonstrate that they care about animals, help build a trust relationship with owners, and also help to calm clients visiting the practice.

For veterinarians to be able to give advice and treat pets they have to have a good relationship with the owners. A good relationship is founded on trust. Establishing trust takes time and determination. Trust is precious: once lost it is hard to regain. Trust is created by showing interest in and concern for a pet in a way that is non-threatening and non-confrontational for the owner, recognising that what is best for the animal has to be balanced against the owner's life-style, capabilities and income, and showing respect for an owner's wishes even if not in complete agreement with them (see *Business considerations*, later).

Best for the practice

> *If we don't give clients what they want and pets what they need, then we risk losing our leadership position to people who are less qualified than we are, or who pass emotion off as fact.*
> Marty Becker, DVM

In 1970, the average veterinary practice in the United States consisted of one veterinarian, very little competition, and a mixed animal practice. It took a community area population of about 10 000 to support that one veterinarian. By 1985, that population catchment area had dropped to one veterinarian per 4000 population (with only about half being pet-owners). Additional services and more client visits per year were required in companion animal practices just to break even with the 'good old days' of lesser competition. In 1985, the American Veterinary Medical Association performed a manpower survey which predicted that, by the end of the century, there would be a 73% increase in the number of private veterinary practitioners, but only a 31% increase in the number of pets. The survey was repeated in 1991: the increase in the number of practitioners was on target, but the companion animal population growth had slowed even more than predicted. The study's conclusion is even more valid now than in 1985:

> *Veterinarians will need to develop and implement practice strategies to realise more of the potential demand for veterinary medical services.*

> *The human–animal bond = the interaction of people and animals in our society*
> *= the profit centre of the future.*

Veterinarians make their living because of the human–animal bond, but most veterinarians do not capitalise upon the potential available. For example, when clients call the veterinarian because they have concerns about the well-being of their animal and want an expert to assist them during their stressful decision time, they *don't* want to be told to stay at home or not worry until tomorrow. They *do* want 'peace of mind', and the successful veterinary practitioner strategically plans to meet this need. Part of this planning is the provision of wellness programmes that increase owner awareness of potential problems and provide systems to prevent these problems from happening.

Well thought through wellness programmes ensure that:

- all patients receive better healthcare on a consistent basis;
- clients encounter fewer crisis episodes due to early problem detection;
- companion animals enjoy a healthier, longer life – which also means a longer and more profitable contact with the practice through increased visits and services;
- there is more effective use of the staff and facilities;
- practice staff members have increased pride in and enjoyment of their work;
- companion animal owners have increased educational contacts with the practice which means clients bond more strongly with 'their' practice, and their knowledge increases in multiple areas, including areas such as dental hygiene, nutrition, parasite control and prevention, behaviour management, reproduction and so on.

Business considerations

The man who will use his skill and constructive imagination to see how much he can give for a dollar, instead of how little he can give for a dollar, is bound to succeed.
Henry Ford

Animal healthcare was once an altruistic community service, but with today's density of veterinarians it is an economic commodity. Many new, hungry, uninformed veterinarians start their practice career by competing on price, rather than by differentiating their practice by providing unmet community needs: even dentistries have become 'quotables' in some communities. This unfortunate attitude is based on a perceived need for personal survival coupled with poor business and leadership skills. Successful veterinary planning centres on meeting the challenges of the marketplace rather than just fulfilling an outdated community service role.

One aspect of the challenge is to define the attitude of the veterinarian to pet-owners. Are they customers or clients?

- A *customer* bargains for commodities. A business exists to provide commodities and is successful if it remains competitive in a dynamic free enterprise system.
- A *client* seeks caring service. A veterinary practice exists to provide services to meet the social contract between society and the healthcare system, which is based on caring, treating, curing, preventing pain, and saving animal life.

The concept that in providing preventive healthcare for companion animals the veterinarian is fulfilling part of his role in the social contract is fundamental to the success of wellness programmes.

The traditional goals of a business are to maximise its profit or market share and, secondarily, to satisfy customer wants. The veterinary hospital seeks to provide quality care for patients in need. While these two approaches are not opposed, in healthcare the order of priorities is provision of quality care, proper compensation to the provider and facility, and the development of a community market niche. There is danger in trying to provide services dependent upon profit motives in a competitive veterinary healthcare marketplace rather than delivering the quality care expected based on the veterinarian's oath. Profit automatically follows a quality healthcare delivery episode, whereas it does not follow an event when the client perceives they have been 'sold' something that wasn't really needed! Remember, *the front door must swing* before any money can be made.

Pet-owners are not 'customers': they have a need to care for their pet in the best possible way. However, many practices unilaterally determine the scope of professional services they will provide, many times failing to offer needed care because of misjudged economic reasoning. They advise their animal owners about the 'minimally adequate' healthcare requirements for their pets, then turn around and scheme how to cross-market additional services to them as if they were just 'customers', so-called bait-and-switch tactics. This is not professional!

Our patients have *needs* not *wants*. Veterinarians are the spokespeople for the health and welfare of animals: they must be able to communicate these needs to the owners. With wellness healthcare, veterinarians are dealing with feelings. Feelings are not just limited to the clients: the desire to fulfil expectations and do a good job, to have pride in caring for the pet while it is in the practice, and to make a personal contribution to a successful outcome are critical elements for staff satisfaction in the healthcare delivery system. The wise veterinarian promotes *team* participation in meeting these wellness and preventive care needs, with the 'team' consisting of staff, client, and the primary veterinary care provider.

Quality care differentiates a caring practice within the community. With the competition and diversity in the United States, those practices which differentiate themselves favourably in the client's mind are successful: the rest, who compete on price, who stay in 'curative medicine', or who cannot release the 'one doctor control' of the practice, are in the 'average masses'. Consider the following:

- In some of the toughest competitive veterinary marketplaces, low-cost vaccination clinics that have started to offer a 'doctor's consultation' (physical exam at a premium price) find that about 75% of their 'economy minded' clients decide to book time with the veterinarian – at a supplemental fee for service.
- At some low-cost spay-neuter clinics, 75% of the 'discount coupon clients' have *declined* to waive needed presurgical laboratory tests – at an additional cost *greater* than the coupon price.
- The superstores in America such as PetsMart and Wal-Mart, even the grocery store down the street, have decided to offer alternatives to the clients of companion animal veterinary practices. They are aggressively competing for the pet healthcare dollar. Some even hire corporations which provide low-cost veterinarians. These 'warehouse vendors' compete on price since they have nothing else to offer the companion animal owner.

When pets in 75% of families are perceived by clients as being members of the family, the animal's *needs* for a higher quality level of concerned preventive veterinary healthcare for enhanced wellness become a major decision factor in caring for the animal.

Providing a balanced healthcare approach ensures our professional position as the guardians of animal health and welfare. The quality-based, communication-rich, caring role of the veterinarian of tomorrow will provide the economic future needed for career-minded new graduates to continue in this healthcare profession with pride.

Conclusion

Pet ecosystem management, optimising health through high levels of preventive health-care, and celebrating and protecting the family–pet–vet bond are the keys to success in veterinary medicine.
Marty Becker, DVM

The progressive veterinary practice understands that client bonding is the secret to success in an overcrowded veterinary community, and marketing of their patient advocacy philosophy feeds this image. Wellness programmes are based on nurturing the family–pet–vet bond. Wellness is not just about vaccinations and parasite evaluation, it is a total 'conception to death' partnership with the companion animal steward. Wellness programmes are necessary to veterinary practice. They are best for pets, best for owners, and best for the practice. The choice is yours! Capitalise on the original covenant as the provider of animal welfare and wellness! Care enough to become committed! Dare to become better than average!

References and further reading

Beck, A.M. and Katcher, A.H. (1983) *Between Pets and People: the Importance of Animals Companionship*. G.P. Putnam's Sons, New York.

Biery, M.J. (1985). Riding and the handicapped. *Veterinary Clinics of North America Small Animal Practice*, **15** (2).

Catanzaro, T. E. (1984) *The Human-Animal Bond in Military Families, The Pet Connection*. CENSHARE, U of MN, MN, pp 341–347.

Friedmann, E., Katcher, A.A., Thomas, S.A. and Lynch, J.J. (1984). Health consequences of pet ownership. In: Kay, W.J. et al (eds) *Pet Loss and Human Bereavement*. Iowa State University Press, New York, p 22–29.

Katcher, A.H. and Friedmann, E. (1980). Potential health value of pet ownership. The compendium on continuing education for the practising veterinarian: the compendium on continuing education for the small animal veterinarian. *New Jersey* **2(2)**, 117–121.

Levinson, B.M. (1975). Pets and environment. In: Anderson, R.S. (ed) *Pet Animals and Society*. Baillière Tindall, London, p 9–18.

Lynch, J.J. (1977). *The Broken Heart: the Medical Consequences of Loneliness*. Basic Books, New York.

Rollin, B.E. (1984). The moral status of animals. In: Kay, W.J. et al (eds) *Pet Loss and Human Bereavement*. Iowa State University Press, New York, p 3–15.

Schneider, R. and Vaida, M.L. (1975). Survey of canine and feline populations: Alameda and Contra Costa Counties, California, 1970. *Journal of the American Veterinary Association* **166**, 481–486.

Youmans, E.G. and Yarrow, M. (1971). Aging and social adaption: A longitudinal study of healthy elderly men. In: Granik, S. and Patterson R.D. (eds) *Human Ageing 11: an Eleven Year Follow-up Biomedical and Behavioural Study*. DHEW Publication number (HSM) 70–9037. U.S. Government Printing Office, Washington D.C., p 95–104.

- American Veterinary Medical Association, manpower survey, G14.
- *The Pet Connection*, CENSHARE, University of Minnesota.
- Pet Placement information, American Veterinary Medical Association (708/925-8070).
- Delta Society (206/226-7357).
- Behavior Management resources, American Animal Hospital Association.
- Pet Owner Survey (1995), American Animal Hospital Association.

Setting up Wellness Programmes

2

Caroline Jevring, Thomas E. Catanzaro

The role of the pet in society has changed. Pets are increasingly regarded as cherished family members. The need from pet-owners for information and products that will help their pet live a healthier and longer life has also changed. Wellness programmes are the veterinarian's response to this need.

Wellness is not new – farm animal veterinarians have been running herd preventive care programmes for years, and most companion animal clinics have some sort of preventive healthcare programmes in place. Unfortunately, these latter have often been rather hit-and-miss affairs.

Wellness programmes go beyond simple preventive healthcare. Preventive healthcare is passive, wellness is active. Owners are actively encouraged to participate in creating an environment for wellness for their pet. The veterinarian, staff, and client work together as a team to provide the best possible care for the pet. In addition, the goal is not simply a healthy pet, but includes quality of life considerations for pet and owner.

Wellness care is practising good medicine: good medicine is profitable. For wellness to work, veterinarians and their clients need structured programmes. Good wellness programmes need planning. Planning is a vital but still rather neglected area of practice management. By planning how to provide your healthcare most effectively you also plan your profit (see Table 2.1).

There are many different programmes that can be established in companion animal practice. These include:
- puppy and dog health
- kitten and cat health
- new pet health
- obesity management
- dental healthcare
- senior healthcare
- care of the pregnant and lactating pet

Note that these programmes differ from the traditional preventive healthcare programmes in that they include all the different aspects of preventive health and ecosystem management for pets of different ages, life-stages, and species.

Table 2.1 Types of wellness programme

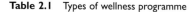

To be successful, wellness programmes require:
- commitment by all the staff to the concepts of total healthcare;
- a proactive rather than a reactive approach to medical management on the part of the practice;
- careful planning and monitoring of results so that programmes are constantly updated and improved;
- constant interaction with, and feedback from, clients.

Wellness programmes run alongside the everyday emergencies and problems of normal practice. They cover all the important life-stages of pets and they interlink with each other so that, for example, an elderly dog that comes in for its annual booster vaccination can be recommended to join the Senior Healthcare Programme, and from there be directed into the Dental Healthcare Programme.

Existing preventive healthcare programmes should be updated and improved before introducing new programmes. Building up a range of wellness programmes step by step, starting by revising and updating the ones you currently have in the practice (such as puppy/kitten vaccination programmes), means that clients get the best from each programme before new ones are introduced, and that the practice does not become overwhelmed with too many new projects at once.

Planning a wellness programme

In this section, broad guidelines for the setting up and management of wellness programmes are given. Other chapters will deal in more detail with specific programmes as relevant.

In planning a wellness programme you need to consider the following questions:
- Why do you want to develop wellness programmes in your practice?
- What are your expectations?
- What are your clients' expectations?
- What are your aims?
- How will you measure success?
- What do you need?
- When and where?
- Who and what?
- How do you develop a protocol?
- What training should your personnel receive?
- How do you market wellness?
- How can you plan for profit?

The exact details differ from programme to programme (see Table 2.2 and Table 2.3, p. 21) but the following approach is a logical and useful basic guide:

Paediatric Healthcare
To work with owners in providing the best possible level of care for their puppy or kitten including recommendations on the importance of correct nutrition, dental prophylaxis, exercise, grooming, disease and parasite control, neutering and behaviour management.

Senior Healthcare
To work with owners in providing the best possible level of care for older animals (over the age of 5–7 years) including control and management of age-related disorders such as organ failure, dental disease, joint and skeletal problems through correct nutrition, exercise and regular screening for early detection of disease.

Dental Prophylaxis
To work with owners in providing the best possible level of dental care through clinical prophylaxis and careful home management. Special attention is given to animals in high risk categories such as toy breeds and brachycephalic breeds.

Behaviour Management
To work with owners to encourage ownership of a well-behaved pet, and to supply expert advice about management and prevention of behaviour problems.

Obesity Management
To educate and inform owners about the risks associated with obesity and how they can help prevent or manage the condition through dietary management and exercise.

Annual Health Checks
To educate and inform owners about the benefits of regular screening of a range of parameters, coupled with advice about correct nutrition and other health maintaining factors to maintain an optimal health status for their pets.

Table 2.2 Aims for specific programmes

Why do you want to develop wellness programmes in your practice?

Why are you starting a new wellness programme? Has new technical information about reducing risk factors for disease recently been published which you want to share with your clients? Are you planning to improve the standard of healthcare offered by the practice? Is this an opportunity to enhance practice income? Do you want to justify the purchase of a new piece of equipment by incorporating its use into a wellness programme? Do you want to utilise staff time more effectively?

What are your expectations?

Commitment to promoting wellness is a long-term action. Establishing wellness programmes in your practice usually represents a change in attitude not only within the practice, but also in how your clients perceive your practice and the services you offer. Changing attitudes takes time. Wellness programmes not uncommonly fail in practice because of unrealistic and over-optimistic expectations about how many people will take up the programmes, and how immediate that response will be. Studies have shown that it can take 5–12 exposures to a new concept before clients will accept it or try it, so it is important not to give up too early.

For example, with a senior programme, although around 40% of your clients' pets may fall into the senior category, probably well under 10% of those eligible will initially be interested in such a programme: on the other hand, with a good recall system you can anticipate an almost 100% response and uptake from your clients on, say, a vaccination programme over the course of the year (see *Marketing*).

What are your clients' expectations?

To get full cooperation from your clients – and their cooperation is largely what the success of wellness programmes depends upon – you need to be absolutely sure that they understand the aims and purpose of each programme. For example, with a puppy health programme you can obviously never guarantee that their puppy will not get sick or even have an accident and die, but by working together with you on the programme they can be assured that they are doing the best they can to ensure a good start in life for their beloved puppy. Similarly, a senior programme cannot stop an elderly cat or dog from dying of old age, but it can help ensure that the last few months or years of life are as comfortable and enjoyable as possible for pet and owner alike.

What are your aims?

By assessing your true reasons for wanting to develop a new programme you gain a clearer view of your aims, and how you can measurably achieve them. In general terms your aims will include:
- to improve the health of the pets in your care, leading to better life quality and greater longevity;
- to give better client service through better pet care;
- to enhance bonding by clients to your practice;
- to improve practice image through practising better veterinary medicine;
- to improve use of staff time and experience;
- to increase staff satisfaction and provide greater opportunity to use their skills and training through greater involvement in healthcare;
- to make more efficient use of practice facilities;
- to increase income for the practice through increased sales of services;
- to celebrate and work with the family–pet–vet bond.

For individual programmes it is helpful to clarify your aims in terms of SMART objectives, i.e.:
- **S**pecific;
- **M**easurable;
- **A**ction-orientated;
- **R**ealistic;
- **T**ime-limited.

An example of a specific SMART objective for a kitten health programme could be:

We aim to improve the general awareness of kitten health and behaviour by offering kitten owners counselling services on such issues as the importance of house-training, vaccination, parasite control, correct nutrition, and behaviour management. The counselling services will take the form of a course of two, weekly 'parties' run by trained staff members and using both internal and external 'experts' plus written handouts, for which owners will pay a small fee. We will promote the parties by word-of-mouth, through posters in the reception area and clinic rooms, and in our newsletter. We will review the success of these parties after the first three months through questionnaires to participants and non-participants that specifically investigate the general level of health and behaviour awareness.

How will you measure success?

Success is a rather arbitrary term but it is important to try and define 'success' for each programme to be able to measure achievement and progress. Measures of success could include:
- *Profit* – e.g. has use of the new laboratory equipment generated enough additional income to pay for itself within the first year? (see *Measuring profitability*, later).
- *Client satisfaction and general awareness of health management issues* – e.g. are clients generally pleased with the senior health programme you run and feel that they are able to contribute in a valuable way to caring for their older pet?
- *Staff satisfaction* – e.g. do staff feel their contribution to pet health is enhanced through being able to run wellness programmes and help owners care better for their pets?
- *Sales of pet foods, dental products, etc.* – e.g. have you achieved the 5% increase in sales of kitten diets/dental chews you wanted within three months?
- *Frequency of cases of preventable disease* – e.g. are pet mouths generally healthier/the incidence of obesity generally lower now than one year ago?

What do you need?

All programmes require the following:

- a committed attitude from the whole practice;
- appropriately trained staff;
- suitable client education materials (information brochures, personalized letters, demonstration models, practice photograph file, illustrative material, etc.);
- appropriate pet health record cards (e.g. one where the weight can be marked on a graph for an obesity programme, or where the major problem areas in a mouth can be illustrated for a dental programme);
- a reminder/recall system (this is much simpler if it is computerised);
- appropriate dietary management;
- cooperation and commitment from clients.

Some programmes may require an investment in certain types of equipment such as a dental scaler and polisher, weighing scales or laboratory equipment (see Table 2.3). As these can be used in many different ways in the practice they represent a worthwhile outlay.

When and where?

For wellness to work it must be integrated into every encounter. This means staff must talk about wellness, give information leaflets freely, and help clients see the importance the practice places on wellness in every contact. For example, when a client phones the practice, the receptionist should automatically check the pet's medical journal to see when it was last vaccinated and its teeth were last checked. All pets should be weighed before a clinical examination and the weight recorded in their journal – this demonstrates the importance of weight in relation to health. Posters and products for sale in the reception area highlight the effective management of common preventive health issues such as parasite control and dental care.

The formal programmes require planning. For example, when are you going to carry out the procedures in the programme? Can the animals be booked in for quieter times in the day such as late morning and early afternoon, perhaps during the middle of the week? Will the animals need to be admitted? How long will the procedures take? Whose time will be involved? Is there a separate room where the support staff member can carry out examinations and client discussions? Should you aim to start this programme in a quieter period of the year?

Different programmes take different amounts of time and may need to be performed in different places. For example, pet behaviour counselling needs around two hours per consultation, a high degree of owner involvement, and often requires a home visit, whereas a senior health programme mainly uses trained support staff time in taking samples and giving much of the general healthcare advice. Be careful not to limit yourself by restricting yourself only to the times immediately convenient to the practice – these are often quiet times *because* they are not convenient to owners.

Paediatric Healthcare
Weighing scales
Model demonstrating dental disease
Toothpaste, toothbrushes
High quality growth diet
Preserved parasite specimens
Diagrams of the lifecycles of external parasites

Senior Healthcare
Weighing scales
Model demonstrating dental disease
Refractometer
Laboratory facilities for haematology and blood biochemistry
Radiographic facilities (ECG; endoscope, etc.)
High quality diet to meet the special nutritional needs of older pets
Preserved parasite specimens

Dental Prophylaxis
Dental scaler and polisher and/or appropriate hand instruments
Toothbrushes and toothpaste
Recommended dental chews
Model demonstrating dental disease
Appropriate high quality (dry) diets

Behaviour management
Appropriate aids to behaviour management
Suitable high quality diet (diet may be a significant factor in some forms of
behavioural abnormality)

Obesity management
Weighing scales
Weight comparison charts
Weight-reducing diet
Weight management diet

Annual Health Checks
Weighing scales
Refractometer
Laboratory facilities for haematology and blood biochemistry
Model of dental disease
Appropriate high quality diets
Preserved parasite specimens

Table 2.3   Suggestions for special equipment checklist

Who and what?

Wellness programmes involve the healthcare team of veterinarian, staff members, and client. For clients to take up the programmes they need to understand the need for and the benefits from using them. They also need continued support in working with the programmes at home. Veterinarians and their staff must be skilled communicators. Unfortunately, this is not always the case.

Veterinarians are trained to speak in 'professional' terms – appropriate if terms are explained, but this occurs too infrequently. Most clients don't understand common terms like FVRCP, DHLAPP, FeLV, FIV, etc., and understand even less about -itis's, -osis's, and -ectomies. A recent survey by the American College of Healthcare Executives showed that 46% of the population did not understand the term 'benign' when used with the word 'cancer'. The result is that clients look to staff to 'translate' and validate what the veterinarian has said. They feel more comfortable discussing concerns with the technician because they don't want to take up the veterinarian's time, or they don't understand the terms he/she uses or, simply, they feel it is easier to talk to the support staff member or receptionist.

Wellness programmes are run by a wellness *team* (Table 2.4). This means they are not the *sole* responsibility of veterinarians, but veterinarians are notorious for trying to do too much themselves and, in turn, not doing enough for each client and pet. In fact, most programmes are ideal for support staff to organise and run. Interestingly, when a staff member becomes a healthcare team member, client communications improve.

In most practices, 80% of client contacts are with the paraprofessional staff. Clients often first express their concerns to a staff member. It is their caring attitude that allows the client to form that all-important 'first impression' and 'practice image', and their knowledge that helps the client make healthcare decisions about needed care for their pet. The greater the client's knowledge of the healthcare needs of their pet, the more likely it is that the animal will receive the needed care. It is thus vital for paraprofessional staff to learn excellent client communication skills.

What training should your personnel receive?

Well-informed and motivated staff – and that includes the veterinarians – are vital to the success of wellness programmes. Motivate staff by involving them in the programmes from the beginning, and empower them to run them according to goals they have helped define.

Teach staff using both internal and invited external speakers. For example, the representative from a vaccine company can describe the use of the vaccines for a vaccine programme, or a veterinary nutritional expert from a pet nutrition company can explain the importance of dietary management in a senior, obesity or kitten programme. Discuss the best laboratory tests to perform with the university experts; invite a pet behaviour specialist to work with the practice. Recommend relevant scientific papers that staff members should read; talk to colleagues who are running similar programmes.

Discuss the application of the new knowledge in practical terms. How can your staff best use this information? What do you want them to say to clients on the phone? In the reception area? In the consulting room? How can this information

Who does the nutritional counselling?
- Are serial weights noted in every medical record?
- Who does the monthly client recall, patient appearance recheck, and monthly sequential weigh-ins?
- Who monitors the client's reorder point for prescription diets?
- Who discusses the home supplementation concerns when the client stops feeding a prescription diet?

Who does the parasite prevention and control counselling?
- Does the practice understand the difference between foggers and a premises eradication guarantee?
- Who actually defines where in the house (floor plan assessments) foggers need to go for most effect versus a total premises plan?
- Who does the follow-up to ensure there is effective elimination?
- Who ensures that the effects of infestation by external and internal parasites are understood by the client?

Who does the dental hygiene counselling?
- Are clients asked to rub the pet's teeth nightly with tuna water (cats) or garlic water (dogs) to see if they tolerate tooth brushing before they commit to more extensive dental care?
- Who discusses the diet and bad breath that results from poor dental hygiene?
- Who cares enough to tell clients that 'red gums mean pain' and explain the healthcare options?

Who does the behaviour management counselling?
- Does it automatically start with the puppy/kitten programme?
- Is house-training assistance given during the first puppy/kitten visit as a value-added service?
- Who spends time listening to the client's needs (85% of clients report a pet behaviour problem)?
- Who schedules short familiarisation times in the clinic, on a weekly basis, to help change the unwanted behaviour?
- Who ensures that the behaviour management ideas are working in the home with all the family members?

Who keeps in touch with the clients?
- Who phones new clients to say 'Welcome to our practice!'?
- Who makes the post-medication dispensing (halfway through treatment) call to ensure that the client does not have questions (and has not stopped the treatment programme or forgotten the recheck appointment)?
- Who makes the post-surgical call, at recovery and again four days after discharge, to ensure the client has no worries?
- Who phones clients who have missed appointments to ask, 'The doctor and I missed you and Fido today, is everything okay at your house?'?

Table 2.4 Defining roles in the practice

be phrased in written client communications? How do you handle client objections? Find out the potential problems and pitfalls and work out how you can overcome them. By finding answers to these questions before you even start, your programme has more chance of success.

Finally, don't forget to praise and reward your staff!

How do you develop a protocol?

A protocol for the programme is essential. It should be clearly and concisely worked out, rehearsed, then modified through team participation. Work through the following questions:

- How do we identify the pet and owner for whom the programme is suitable?
- How do we explain the benefits to the owner and gain their commitment to the programme?
- How will the owner participate? What do they do at home, e.g. dietary management, teeth-cleaning, behaviour training?
- What is the role of the veterinary surgeon?
- What is the role of the support staff?
- What is the role of external experts?
- How do we recommend healthcare products and their use?
- How do we use educational and support materials?

Medical and treatment decisions lie with the veterinarian, but support staff will have valuable suggestions on how to make the programme run smoothly and effectively. A trial run of the programme in its entirety using a colleague's or cooperative client's pet can iron out any problems before it is introduced into the practice.

How do you market wellness?

The services that veterinarians think their clients don't want, most clients WON'T want. Why? Because they don't KNOW the services are available.
Dooley, 1992

Marketing is the analysis, planning, implementation and control of carefully formulated programmes which are designed to encourage and build a productive and profitable relationship between an organisation, such as a veterinary practice, and its target market, a specific group or groups of animal owners.

Market research to establish the need for a programme is an essential starting point. Discussing successful programmes with colleagues in other practices can be an encouraging pointer but most important of all is that you ask your clients what *they* want, and *listen* to their replies. It is *not* adequate to rely only on your own feelings about what clients do and don't want: you do not perceive pet health as your clients do.

Clients usually have fairly clear ideas about what they want for their pets. Interestingly, whatever you *choose to believe* about your clients you will find happening with them. Thus, if *you choose* to offer a minimum service because *you believe* clients don't really care about their animals and do not want to pay much for treatment, you will attract those clients who only want minimal service. The caring pet-owners will go to those veterinarians who believe their clients want the best for their animals, and who offer and strongly recommend this level of service.

This observation is amply borne out through various management studies. For example, Wutchiett's Well-Managed Practices, which represent some of America's best run and efficient practices, have the following characteristics:

- income of over $250 000 per vet per year;
- 3.2 support staff per veterinarian;
- 1270 active clients per vet.

New figures from a survey in 1997 of over 37 000 clients through an educational grant from Pfizer Animal Health gave the following client profile:

- 80% of clients are female: women are the caregivers for the entire family, including pets;
- 76% own dogs;
- 47% own cats;
- 65% live within a 5 mile radius of the practice;
- the average owner spends $173.20 per year but 51% spend over $200 per year;
- on average clients visit their practice 5.1 times per year, of which three are for veterinary procedures, the remainder being for purchase of healthcare products;
- 89% selected the practice originally for its location and/or referral by friends.

How can you use information like this to promote healthcare effectively and profitably in your practice?

The problems of marketing services

A wellness programme is an example of a professional service. A service is defined as *any activity or benefit that one party can offer to another that is essentially intangible and does not result in the ownership of anything.* This intangibility makes marketing wellness programmes especially challenging.

It is important for practice members to understand the concepts behind marketing wellness. They are *not* simply selling a procedure or product – they are selling a whole package of wellness care.

Start by clearly defining what the service is: a practice does not sell just a neuter, for example, but a healthcare package that includes:

- a clinical examination by a veterinarian;
- an operation which will modify undesirable sexually-related behaviour, reduce the risk of certain malignant tumours developing (depending on species and age at time of operation), and prevent undesirable reproduction;
- promotion of a healthier and longer life for the animal concerned because its frustrated sexuality is no longer a problem for the pet or the owner (e.g. through behaviour-related problems such as territorial aggression, wandering, and unwanted pregnancy);
- promotion of a healthier and longer life for the animal concerned because the chances of developing serious diseases such as testicular cancer, pyometra or mammary neoplasia later in life are reduced or eradicated;
- reassurance for the responsible owner that they are doing the best thing for their pet.

Similarly, the sale of professional healthcare products by a trained staff member confers a number of integral advantages:

- It helps the pet-owner make an informed decision about which healthcare products are best for the pet.
- It guarantees a professional standard of product.
- It encourages the client to bond more strongly with the practice through repeat sales of products.
- It improves pet health.
- It provides reassurance for the responsible owner that they are doing the best thing for their pet.

Target marketing in healthcare has three clear steps:

- *making the client aware that there are many factors which can influence their pet's health;*
- *letting the client clearly understand that the veterinary profession – and, more specifically, your practice – now has ways of helping to maintain the pet in optimal health throughout its life by creating a safe, healthy environment for it;*
- *clearly informing the client that the practice team has several ways in which they can provide these services and meet the need to maintain wellness.*

Informing the client

The response to any programme depends partly on how enthusiastically you and your staff market it. For example, a targeted letter to clients alone will probably give a less than 10% response rate, whereas a letter plus a phone call from a trained member of staff can boost the response to a much higher level. Some or all of the following methods of promoting a programme to your clients can be considered:

- Train your staff to identify opportunities to talk to clients about the new service.
- Follow up with personal contact to ensure home care is carried out correctly.
- Make a display in the practice using promotional literature and posters.
- Target mail information to clients.
- Use reminders (written and telephone).
- Print articles in the practice newsletter.
- Encourage features on local TV and radio stations: local newspapers may be interested in a brief article promoting the concepts of preventive health.

Promoting the benefits

The promotion of the service needs to be in the form of the BENEFITS of the service rather than the promotion of the service itself. Through promotion, the sale should be made at the programme level rather than at an individual service level, promoting the total health programme rather than a single vaccination or bag of dog food.
McCurnin, 1988

As an exercise, list the benefits of a programme to the practice, the staff, the clients and the pets. This serves two functions:
- It clarifies why you want this programme and what you hope to get out of it.
- It helps your staff identify the benefits they should discuss with the client, which is how the programme is best promoted.

First and foremost, the animals in your care benefit with improved life quality and expectancy. Periodontal disease, for example, affects more than 85% of animals over the age of 3 years. It can be effectively managed by a rigorous control programme combining routine clinical examinations and home care, ideally starting from the puppy or kitten's first visit to the surgery.

Around 25% of dogs in the UK are obese and are thus at risk of developing locomotor disorders and joint disease, diabetes mellitus, circulatory problems and certain types of neoplasia. Obesity can be prevented through counselling owners about the seriousness of the disease, and instigating better feeding habits for their pets.

In the United States, behaviour problems are the primary reason for euthanasia of dogs between weaning and maturity. In the UK most of the cases treated could have been avoided had the pet been purchased from a better source and socialised properly with its own kind and people during critical weeks of development. Raising breeder and client awareness of the importance of having a well behaved, well socialised pet through running behaviour advisory programmes can help to prevent unnecessary deaths.

Pet-owners benefit from wellness programmes by having a happier, healthier pet. Through increased awareness of the risks that can lead to disease, they can make more informed decisions about their pet's health and, in the long term, save money on the potentially high cost of treatments of preventable conditions.

The practice benefits in many ways from wellness programmes. For example, staff gain more satisfaction from practising better medicine and enjoy the increased responsibility from more personalised client contact. Practice profit can significantly increase through more productive use of trained staff time plus sales of quality health products. These profits can, at least in part, be ploughed back into the practice for further development and improvement of client services.

'Selling' healthcare

Veterinary practices 'sell' only one thing – peace of mind for the client. Clients are not well informed consumers of veterinary healthcare services. They do not understand the levels of quality and training that are so variable between the suppliers available. As a profession, we have not greatly helped this situation: we still deal in 'quotables' on a daily basis. However, communicating to win is not selling a fixed service or product, it is letting people buy what they seek. Look at the world around you. People are not sold newspapers, they buy information (or comics, or sports). You don't want to be sold circus tickets – you want to buy the thrills and entertainment. When someone parks a new car in their driveway, the first statement is 'Look at the neat car I just *bought* …' but when something goes wrong, the phrase becomes, 'Look at the lemon they *sold* me!'.

We must learn to fulfil *client* needs and wants through using the skill of listening – something we are not very good at. Opportunities often arise, for example, during the physical examination of a patient, and these must then be prioritised into the care plan.

Communicating to win – that is, encouraging buying not pushing selling – has four basic steps that any practice can learn to follow:

1 Identify the *pre-existing* condition that needs attention and that is a concern to the owner. This could be anything from a problem with 'wind' to a suspicious growth.
2 Teach the client about the changes in the veterinary profession that now enable us to address the condition.
3 With caring and enthusiasm, offer your practice's programme to address the client's concern (patient's problem).
4 After the client replies, validate the response, regardless of what it is, and set the expectation for the next encounter. Whether the client has opted for full service, partial care, deferred service, or simply waived the care, they must feel comfortable with their decision if you want them to return to the practice another time. Return visits make a greater net for the

practice than the search for new clients, so to establish the expectation for their next visit is part of the 'comforting' action. If the dental decision was '… not today …' assign a technologist to the client/patient and set expectations for their telephone follow-up to ensure the 'red gums (red = pain)' are resolved. You accept them and their decision, and you want to see them again!

Be ready for the client to ask the basic buying questions when you explain the treatment or management options: What is it? Why do I need it? How much is it? Is it really needed now? What is the value to me? Remember, the client bases most decisions on the *emotion* of the moment, while the average veterinary practice addresses the *logic* of the need. Logic seldom answers the emotional need, nor does the 'tincture of time' brush-off. The pet-owner wants to know how much you care, not how much you know.

Clients are given options and are allowed to select from these (see Box 2.1): they are encouraged to 'buy' what they think they can afford. Cheaper alternatives are not offered until the client asks for them, but the 'options' must clarify the significance of diminished diagnostics, or desired healthcare effects. Remember, clients prefer to 'buy' and hate being 'sold' so train the practice team to 'sell' *only* peace of mind, freedom from fears, or psychological comfort while allowing the client to 'buy' products and services to their heart's content! Naturally, the client's economy dictates how much they can afford during any one visit, so one aspect of the support staff's role can be to maintain contact with the client and get them to return on a regular, frequent basis for some of the other care needed.

Early on, clients need to know that you treat the whole animal in relation to the whole family, not just a part of the animal, and that they can trust you to differentiate the needs of the animal from those of the practice. For instance, a pre-anaesthesia laboratory profile is a professional need to ensure there isn't something going on that cannot be seen which may cause anaesthetic complications.

Box 2.1 *Two 'yes' options*

The two yes options is a philosophy of providing needed care as a patient advocate rather than expecting the client to have attended veterinary school to be able to select from the options offered. Pre-anaesthetic laboratory screening is a good example:

'Ms Smythe, we need to do a pre-anaesthetic blood screen before Muffy's general anaesthesia, and we can either do the minimal level or an annual baseline. The minimal will give us a look at the packed red blood cell volume for oxygen carrying capacity, the total protein for hydration needs, and the blood urea nitrogen for basic kidney function and the kidney's ability to eliminate toxins. The annual baseline is a full chemistry panel which gives us more in-depth information about the current wellness of most of the body organs. If Muffy becomes ill in the next year or two, it gives us a wellness baseline to check against for changes. Which would you prefer today, Ms Smythe?'

How can you plan for profit?

If you can't measure it, you can't manage it!

Profit is defined as the difference between the level of income earned and the costs incurred in earning it over a particular period of time. From a financial management point of view it is most effective to treat each wellness programme as a profit centre in its own right. This means carefully measuring the costs and the income from each programme to monitor the profitability accurately. This is illustrated in general terms in the equation below.

Profit	**=**	**Income**	**–**	**Costs**
		Client uptake of services and products		Planning time
				Staff training
		Continued, long-term use of specific products		Staff time
				Employing an expert
		Uptake of other services and products		Promotional literature
				Mailing costs
				Special equipment
				Professional health products
				Marketing costs

Trained support staff can run wellness programmes. This has several advantages:
- It encourages support staff to indulge their creativity and imagination.
- It encourages support staff to take responsibility for the profitability of their own income centres.
- It gives more job satisfaction through greater involvement, and measurable outcomes.
- It enhances practice profitability.
- It releases the veterinary surgeons for procedures more suited to their skills and training.
- Clients are more willing to talk freely to staff members and are more likely to ask them about other services available for the better health of their animals.

Pricing wellness programmes

Pricing wellness programmes is often a major stumbling block to their establishment because practices are not sure how to measure and express the benefits of the programme to themselves or to their clients. Consider the following:

- The fee charged should accurately reflect the time and expertise involved.
- In some cases it may be worth charging a lower programme fee because of the high likelihood that the patient will need further treatment (for example, a relatively low cost geriatric examination is likely to generate money from dentals, 'lumpectomies', blood work and so on).
- Calculate all the costs involved and express this as a package.
- Explain the *benefits* of the programme and how it can help the health of the pet to convince interested owners of the *value* of the fee. Remember, only 20% of people make a buying decision based on price alone: 80% of people consider value and benefits as well.

Summary

1 Planning programmes for pet wellness is challenging and rewarding.
2 Wellness benefits pet health through helping owners create an environment for good health and helps bond clients to the practice.
3 Practising wellness medicine is practising better medicine.

References and further reading

Bush, B.M. (1992) Obesity in small animals, its causes, diagnosis and treatment. *Veterinary Practice Clinical Review* **1**(6), 1–7.

Catanzaro, T.E. (1998) *Income Centre Management. Building the Successful Veterinary Practice: Programs & Procedures* (Chap. 4, Vol. 2). Iowa State University Press, Ames, Iowa.

Dooley, D.R. (1992). Negativity gets you nowhere. *Veterinary Economics* **July**, 46–49.

Emily, P. and Penman, S. (1990). *Handbook of Small Animal Dentistry*. Pergamon Press, Oxford.

Hodgkins, E.M. (1990). Bringing wellness to companion animals. *Partners in Practice* **3**(3). PO Box 148, Topeka, Kansas.

Jevring, C. (1995). *Managing a Veterinary Practice*. W.B. Saunders, London, p 118–130.

McCurnin, D.M. (1988). *Veterinary Practice Management*. J.B. Lippincott, Philadelphia.

Myers, W.S. (1997). Who are your clients? *Veterinary Economics* **May**, 46–53.

Myers, W.S. (1997). What do clients want? *Veterinary Economics* **June**, 40–49.

Wutchiett, C. (1994). You can increase your practice revenue. *Veterinary Economics* **September**, 40–44.

Care of the Young Pet

3

Sarah Heath

For many owners the first encounter they have with a veterinary practice is at the time of the new pet's first vaccination. Already the veterinarian has lost the chance to offer advice on pet selection to the prospective owner, and a mismatch may have occurred. At least practice members can give complete coverage of all aspects of puppy or kitten care including advice on house-training, correct nutrition, and exercise requirements. Or can they? Practice members surely know how to encourage clients to make full use of the services that the practice has to offer. Or do they?

For too long veterinary practices have been the place to take an animal when it starts to fall apart rather than the place to go to prevent that happening in the first instance. Owners need to be encouraged to approach practice members with *any* problems and queries related to their pet, not just those of a medical nature. If the profession fails to provide new owners with the help and support that they need then owners will simply go elsewhere and ask less well informed people who may give dangerously unreliable advice.

Total pet care takes time and commitment but should not be viewed as an optional extra: it is a vital part of small animal practice.

The first visit by the young pet and its owner to the veterinary practice is one of the most important visits of its life, but in many practices it is simply fitted into the slot between removing stitches and squeezing anal glands. Not only is this crucial first visit a time to help owners with their concerns and teach them about pet wellness, it is also a time to start to build the relationship between pet-owner and practice that may last the pet's lifetime and beyond. Five or ten minute appointments are simply not adequate for transmitting the amount of information that is needed, plus the interest and personal concern. The alternatives include:

- longer first and second vaccination appointments;
- 'new pet' clinics offering additional appointments to discuss aspects of new pet care;
- puppy parties and kitten information evenings.

Some of the information given during the first consultation should only be given by the veterinary surgeon, but a great deal can be dealt with by the other members of the practice staff. A team approach to pet care is recommended because it frees the veterinary surgeon for purely 'veterinary' work, enables veterinary nurses to use their training and experience to much greater effect, and also serves to enhance practice image. Veterinary nurses are eminently well qualified to provide the 'new pet' clinics and to run the puppy parties and kitten information evenings.

Only a fraction of the information that is imparted verbally during consultations is retained by clients. It is therefore essential to use a combination of communication methods to ensure that vital information concerning the health and welfare of the new pet is not simply forgotten.

Possible methods of communication include:
- face-to-face communication in the consulting room;
- leaflets and pamphlets in the vaccination pack;
- posters in the reception area;
- books and video tapes for hire or sale.

The first visit that the young puppy or kitten pays to the veterinary practice will shape that animal's relationship with the veterinary profession for the rest of its life. Fearful behaviour in the consulting room accounts for countless hours of wasted time, unnecessarily high levels of stress for all concerned and, in many cases, the risk of injury. The first visit for the pet should create positive associations. Learning that the veterinary practice is a fun and happy place to be is a vital lesson and one that will reap benefits later. Play, fuss and give the pet treats during the first physical examination to reward compliant behaviour. Give the first vaccination quietly with the minimum of fuss. If the pet is particularly apprehensive then it is better to delay the vaccination for a couple of days and work on increasing the pet's confidence and its positive associations with the practice rather than plough on and risk the negative experience of a traumatic first visit.

Encourage owners to come to the practice between appointments and bring the pet in to help it learn that the practice is a fun place to visit. This applies both to puppies and kittens. Conditioning kittens to visit the veterinary practice and to ride in the car are very simple measures which are rarely even considered by new cat-owners but which can make life much less traumatic later on. Leave bowls of food treats (both canine and feline) on the front desk; when a client comes into the practice the receptionist can offer the owner a friendly and welcoming smile and the pet a tasty treat! Entering the practice soon becomes a positive experience and when the pet 'wants' to come to the vet the owner is far more likely to visit. The more visits that are made, the stronger the relationship between practice and client and the greater the indirect benefits through increased sales of merchandise, uptake of services and good word of mouth publicity.

In many of the larger practices it is possible that the new pet encounters a range of people when it visits. This may be an advantage if each staff member takes the time to introduce themselves to both pet and owner in a positive manner, and if each has read the pet's record card carefully. The risk is that important information may not be given to the owner because of the misconception that someone else has covered it! For example, some owners may get advice about dentistry and worming twice but never receive any guidance about correct nutrition. In order to avoid this situation, the practice should formulate a checklist of topics to be covered with each new owner which is attached to the animal's records (Tables 3.1 and 3.2). Each topic is marked off as it is discussed and the next member of staff who talks with that owner will know what remains to be covered. At the end of the second vaccination appointment the owner can be offered an appointment at the New Pet clinic and the veterinary nurse can see at a glance which topics she needs to discuss in order to complete the information package.

Producing a new owners' information pack can help to ensure that no ends are left untied, and naming a member of staff as the 'new owner contact' you reassure owners that they can always phone or call in for additional help and support.

Health topics
   Vaccination and need for annual boosters
   Internal and external parasite control
   Nutrition
   Dental care
   Nail care
   Neutering

Management topics
   Housing (making the home safe)
   Identification
   Grooming
   Bathing
   Exercise (including suitable equipment, e.g. collars, leads, etc.)
   Pet insurance

Behaviour topics
   House-training
   Handling exercises
   Socialisation and habituation
   Understanding natural canine behaviour and communication
   Effects of neutering on behaviour
   Chewing
   Digging
   Appropriate toys and play
   Appropriate use of rewards and discipline
   Prevention of specific behaviour problems
   Use of indoor pens
   Puppy parties and playgroups
   Training

Table 3.1 An example of a checklist for new puppies

Health topics
Vaccination and need for annual boosters
Internal and external parasite control
Nutrition
Dental care
Claw care
Neutering

Management topics
Housing (making the home safe)
Identification
Indoor/outdoor life-style
Grooming
Pet insurance

Behaviour topics
Use of litter tray
Handling exercises
Socialisation and habituation
Understanding natural feline behaviour and communication
Effects of neutering on behaviour
Appropriate toys and play
Appropriate use of rewards and discipline
Prevention of specific behaviour problems
Kitten information evening
Training

Table 3.2   An example of a checklist for new kittens

Feeding the new puppy or kitten

Nutrition is a subject that has received a great deal of attention in recent years, but it is still an area which causes pet-owners confusion. Few owners want to prepare their own food for their pets and the majority believe that feeding their puppy or kitten simply involves picking a pet food from the supermarket shelf. Teaching owners about the nutritional requirements of their new pet is often helped by drawing parallels with humans and explaining that, just as a new baby is fed different foods from a teenager or an elderly person, so their pet will require a changing diet to provide the correct nutrition at the varying stages of its development. All of the major pet food manufacturers have invested a great deal in the promotion of the 'life cycle' diets, and veterinary practices are in an ideal position to market and advise on these diets.

Specific information on the dietary requirements of puppies and kittens is available elsewhere but some key points to consider are:

- *Quality and digestibility of nutrients* – many kitten diarrhoeas resolve simply by changing from a supermarket brand to a premium brand. The ingredients are much better quality, enhancing nutrient availability and digestibility.
- *Calcium and phosphorus ratio* – balanced premium quality rations designed for growth contain the correct balance of minerals for healthy skeletal growth. Owners do not need to give supplements. Abnormal skeletal growth may occur when growing pets are fed an unbalanced homemade ration.
- *Energy and protein levels* – owners of large breed dogs are often afraid their puppies will grow too fast on growth-type foods and develop problems such as hip dysplasia. It is important to explain that most animals eat to satisfy their energy requirements: by feeding a balanced premium quality diet, owners ensure that when the pet has fulfilled its energy requirements it simultaneously has taken in the correct amounts of protein, minerals and vitamins.
- *Dry diets for cats* – feeding dry diets to cats has been associated with urinary tract disease, especially the formation of bladder struvite in cats. Although most manufacturers of dry cat kibble have reduced the amount of magnesium in their diets, they have not all used ingredients that ensure the cat will produce an acid urine, which is critical to preventing the formation of struvite. Owners should understand that only veterinary-recommended premium cat diets satisfy these requirements, and also that urinary tract disease in cats is multi–factorial, of which correct diet is only one of the factors.

Some other common issues are dealt with in Chapter 5.

Internal and external parasite control

New owners are often very concerned about the control of parasites in and on their new pet, especially where there are young children in the family. They are aware of zoonotic hazards but usually have a rather hazy idea of the risks involved. Owners should be informed in such a way that they are given a balanced and realistic view of the more common parasites of pets. Present a practical approach to parasite control and encourage them to purchase good quality, effective products from the practice. Explain that this is one area of healthcare which will involve regular and frequent medication. Support verbal instructions with clear written information. The manufacturers of parasiticides usually provide good client brochures describing their products and how to use them.

Internal parasites

Give new owners plenty of information about tapeworms and roundworms to answer the common questions they may be reluctant to ask. These include:

How does my dog or cat become infected?

The life-cycles of parasites can be confusing and difficult to understand, and many owners find it helpful to be given diagrams that simplify the process. These can also be useful in illustrating links between parasites, for example *Dipylidium caninum* and the flea or *Taenia taeniaformis* and small rodents. This also encourages vigilance with parasite control. Similarly, information about the routes of infection for the roundworms clarifies for owners the need for regular worming of young puppies and kittens, clearing up of dog faeces from parks and roadside verges, and regular worming of outdoor cats who have access to the faeces of other cats and to other animals or birds who may be latently infested.

What are the signs of infestation?

Owners will ask how they can tell if their pet is infested with internal parasites. It is important to emphasise that parasite control is preventative – it is not a case of waiting for signs of infestation before treating. The presence of tapeworm segments around the anus, for example, can very easily be overlooked, especially in the cat that is continually grooming and reinfecting itself. Signs such as irritation around the anus and digestive disturbances may not become apparent until the parasitic burden is fairly significant.

Are my family at risk?

Media attention to blindness in children caused by migrating ascarids has done much to heighten fears about the zoonotic potential of internal parasites of the cat and dog. Although it is not a cause for hysteria, it is true that hazards exist. People can easily pick up roundworm eggs on their hands from soil, faeces and contaminated objects in the environment and even from the pets themselves (although as it takes approximately two weeks for eggs to reach the point where they can infect the host, pets probably form the lowest source of risk). Children are particularly likely to transfer these eggs to their mouths. The eggs hatch inside the person's digestive system, and the immature worms can migrate around the body causing damage en route. Serious effects are extremely rare. On average there are only two recorded cases of *Toxacara*-related disease per million people each year but even that is two too many. *T. cati*, the tapeworm of cats, has not been associated with human illness to anywhere near the same extent as *Toxacara canis*.

Humans can also become infested with either dog or cat tapeworms if they accidentally swallow a flea which is carrying the tapeworm. However the zoonotic potential of tapeworms is much lower than that of roundworms.

How can they be controlled?

Many owners are surprised at the frequency of dosing required with anthelmintic preparations to keep their pets worm free. Sending worming reminders at two to three month intervals is impractical and owners should develop their own reminder system, such as noting the date when worming treatment is due on their calendar. The months fly by very quickly and owners find that it is remarkably easy to forget the task of worming the family pet.

External parasites

(The management and control of the most important external parasites is covered in more detail in Chapter 11.)

Although dogs and cats can become infested with a range of external parasites including lice, ticks and mites, by far the most common of the external parasites is the flea. Owners are often embarrassed to admit that their pet 'has fleas' and there is a perceived stigma attached to the subject. Being frank and open about the topic as soon as the owner acquires a pet should help them to feel at ease asking for advice. Once again, taking the time to explain the life-cycle of the flea will help owners better to understand the methods of control. Diagrams can be helpful. It is essential to get over the message that fleas do not spend their entire life-cycle on the pet, as lack of environmental treatment in a flea control programme is one of the most common reasons for failure. It is important to inform owners of the phenomenal reproductive ability of the flea and explain that flea control is an ongoing responsibility for *all* pet owners. Owners need to be able to recognise a flea when they see one and also to identify flea dirt, both on their pets and around the house. In the case of cats especially, flea bite allergy is a very common cause of skin disease and many owners find it hard to accept that their cat has fleas, especially when they can see no evidence of them on their pet.

A practice leaflet that gives answers to the commonly asked questions and reassures owners that the presence of fleas is not a sign of poor hygiene is an easy way of getting the message across. Owners need information about the route of transmission, the signs of flea infestation, both on themselves and their pet as well as in the house, and the methods of control, both on the pet and in the environment. As with the control of internal parasites, owner education is the key to success.

Grooming and bathing

Owners of long haired breeds are aware of the need for regular grooming but it is important that all clients appreciate that grooming is not an option but a necessity. Puppy owners are more likely to take grooming seriously since most cat owners believe that the cat should be able to take care of its own coat, especially if it is short haired. Explain to owners that grooming is not only related to management of the coat – it also assists in the early detection of skin disease and has a role in social communication. Involve as many members of the family as possible and encourage the establishment of a regular time for daily grooming. The kittens of long haired cats must be introduced to the grooming as early as possible to avoid later problems with knotting and matting of the coat. Many veterinary practices stock combs and brushes, and a staff member should be able to offer specific advice about what is best for any coat type. It is this sort of advice that sets the veterinary practice apart from the pet shop and will encourage clients to purchase their goods from you.

Puppy owners are more likely to ask about bathing their pet than cat owners but it is sensible to discuss this aspect of coat care with all new owners. Advise them to bath their pet only when it is necessary to do so, for example when the coat is particularly dirty or the young pup or kitten has rolled in something unmentionable, as frequent bathing using shampoos can damage the coat. Selection of a suitable shampoo is important: owners should select one that is balanced to the pH of the animal's skin. Although cats are generally far less tolerant of being bathed than dogs it is possible to condition a young kitten to accept the process. Research in the United States has shown that regular bathing of the family cat can significantly reduce the risks of the pet contributing to problems of allergy or asthma; some owners may therefore benefit from teaching their kitten that bath time is fun.

Dental care (see also Chapter 6)

Periodontal disease is a common problem for dogs and cats, and one where prevention is certainly better than cure. Regular routine dental care such as daily tooth brushing for puppies and kittens is vital to prevent dental disease. Many owners, especially cat owners, find the concept of brushing their pet's teeth strange! However, if the puppy or kitten is introduced early to this routine it soon becomes an accepted part of life. The practice can encourage owners by stocking toothpastes and brushes as well as appropriate chew toys. Take time to teach the owner how to brush the pet's teeth. Use the opportunity during the demonstration to highlight the other strand to dental care: attention to diet.

Exercise recommendations

Puppy owners know they need to exercise their pet but many are unsure of how much exercise is required and how best to provide it. Explaining why dogs need to exercise and why they need to play can help owners to understand their role in their pet's development. Exercise is needed in order to allow the dog to express normal canine behaviours, such as exploring, following scent trails and even hunting. It also helps to improve co-ordination, keeps the body in trim, and keeps the mind alert and active. In addition, exercise helps to reinforce training and provides an opportunity for the development of the pet–owner relationship. Teaching young puppies how to play and providing them with suitable toys and games is a vital aspect of caring for them. Owners need to learn what is acceptable in terms of play: for example, they should avoid activities that encourage jumping up, rough and tumble, and tug of war, as these can lead to behavioural problems later on. There is a great deal of information available to new puppy owners on exercise and play, and the veterinary practice can help to disseminate this information effectively by stocking books and toys at the practice and giving additional advice via the new pet clinic.

Cats also need the opportunity to engage in normal behaviour patterns. Formal exercise is not usually associated with cats, although some owners do take their pets for a walk using harnesses and leads. The cat usually sees to its own exercise and play needs by spending time outdoors, and owners supplement their activity with toys around the house. When the cat is kept entirely indoors there is an an increase in the cat owner's responsibility to provide for the physical and mental needs of the cat in the form of toys and games. Teaching owners how to play with their cat may sound unnecessary but unfortunately many owners are unfamiliar with the natural behaviour patterns of the species and the provision of information about suitable toys and activities should be part of the practice's service to new pet-owners.

Housing

Deciding on whether the new pet is going to live an indoor or outdoor life is a very personal matter. Traditionally the dog is an indoor pet whose access to outdoors is under the control of the owner, whilst the cat is more independent, choosing for himself where he wants to spend his time. Of course this is not always the case – some people feel perfectly at ease keeping their dog outside in a kennel, or their kitten permanently indoors. Whichever method of accommodation is selected, owners must be able to provide for the animal's needs in terms of physical requirements and mental well-being. Dogs and cats need the opportunity to express their natural behaviours and this need has to be reconciled with the practical considerations of ensuring that the home is a safe environment in which to bring up a young puppy or kitten. Veterinary practices can help by giving practical advice about the design of kennels and outdoor cat runs, the options for allowing a cat a semi-outdoor existence via cat flaps, and how to enrich the life of an indoor cat. These issues are best covered in new pet clinics or new owner information evenings.

Vaccination (see Chapter 7)

Vaccination of pets, both a primary course and ongoing boosters, is important for reasons of disease prevention and socialisation. Owners need to understand which diseases the vaccination programme covers and why, and they should also be told that a vaccination is not a guarantee. Timing of the vaccination programme is crucial for disease prevention and the prevention of behavioural problems through socialisation and habituation (see Chapter 9).

Neutering

Responsible pet ownership includes birth control. New owners need to be provided with the relevant information to make an informed decision about breeding from the family pet (see Chapter 8).

Regular health checks

Having provided the new owner with a wealth of information on the care of their new pet, the practice needs to foster a close and ongoing relationship with the client. This is achieved by highlighting the need for regular health check-ups and emphasising the role of prevention in the management of the animal's health. Owners should be encouraged to visit the practice regularly, both for health checks with the veterinary surgeon and for development checks by the veterinary nurse. In addition owners can monitor their pet's health themselves. Teaching owners how to carry out basic health examinations of eyes, ears, mouth, feet and skin can vastly improve the chances of detecting health problems at an early stage. Similarly, owners can learn to monitor their pet's behaviour and be encouraged to discuss any concerns, however trivial they may seem, with the practice staff. Dealing early with inappropriate behaviour is always easier than coping with an established behaviour problem later.

Socialisation and habituation (see Chapter 9)

Preventing the development of behaviour problems is a vital aspect of caring for the young pet. Although the responsibility for starting a successful programme of socialisation and habituation rests with the breeder it is the new owners who will continue the process. All too often the emphasis of caring for a new puppy or kitten rests on providing for its physical needs, and the importance of the animal's psychological development is overlooked.

This is especially true for kittens (Fig. 3.1). The main reason for this is that lack of socialisation in dogs can have very dramatic effects on the animal's behaviour and, due to the different way in which we live with our dogs, those behavioural changes have a more direct impact on our lives. On the whole, dogs do not have the same opportunities as cats to escape from situations: we are all aware of the aggression shown by unsocialised animals who find themselves cornered in fear-inducing situations. Most cats find it easier to run away and, until recently, most

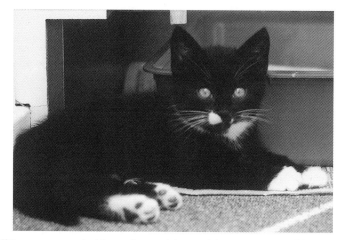

Fig. 3.1 Kitten owners need advice on litter training, nutrition, parasite control, behaviour and reproductive management. © Ann F. Stonehouse.

owners would have accepted this aloofness as normal behaviour. However, with the increasing popularity of the cat there is increasing demand that it lives up to expectations as a companion animal. Owners are distressed if their relationship with their cat is less than ideal: problems are even more apparent in the indoor cat where the animal is expected to live in close proximity with the family with limited opportunity for escape. Unsocialised cats do not make rewarding companions. Paying attention to socialisation and habituation is just as important for kittens as it is for puppies.

New owners should appreciate that puppies and kittens must learn to live within a human society. Socialisation increases their acceptance of other animals, both of their own and of other species, and habituation enables them to cope with the environmental stimuli that they encounter. Exposing the young animal to as wide a range of people, animals and experiences as possible increases the likelihood of having a confident, well adjusted and sociable family pet. Failure to do so not only threatens the mental well-being of the animal, but increases the risk of the development of fear-related behaviour problems that can have dramatic effects later in life. Such a vital part of the animal's development cannot be left to chance: owners should be encouraged to view the socialisation and habituation of their pet as a long-term project. It can be helpful to provide new owners with a socialisation and habituation checklist and encourage them to make a concerted effort to introduce their pet to as many of the situations on the list as possible. For example, instead of simply ensuring that the puppy or kitten meets men, women, and children, introduce people with beards, glasses, walking sticks and distinctive gaits as well! Taking the puppy to a range of places such as the pub, the park and the town is good basic habituation, but diversifying to include the railway station, the football match, the school fete and the local gymkhana will further develop its confidence.

A possible socialisation and habituation checklist which can be expanded and developed to suit puppies or kittens is given in Table 3.3. Obviously not all of these situations and experiences will be relevant to both species.

Although the *range* of experiences and individuals that the pet encounters is important, the *nature* of those experiences is also significant. If the circumstances in which the puppy or kitten meets new people are traumatic then the process will be counterproductive. For example, although it is often beneficial to have a puppy raised in the midst of a chaotic family it can be detrimental if the chaos is such that the puppy is constantly exposed to such a high noise level and activity level that it is unable to rest (Fig. 3.2). Exposure to children is a great advantage to the puppy or kitten unless the children are allowed to maul the animals without any degree of supervision, when the process will undoubtedly backfire. Positive and controlled introductions are the key to success and the well-timed delivery of rewards will assist in establishing good associations with new experiences.

If at any time during the process of socialisation and habituation the puppy or kitten shows a fearful reaction it is very important that owners know how to behave. They must remain calm and not over-react. The owner must appear unworried by the stimulus and not try to reassure the animal as it may well interpret such reassurance as a fear reaction on the part of the owner. It is essential that no animal is ever forced to approach a novel item as this will only draw

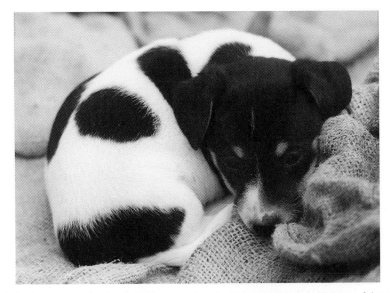

Fig. 3.2 A new puppy needs plenty of time to sleep. Explaining the care requirements of the new, young family member is an important part of a client puppy/kitten programme. © Ann F. Stonehouse.

Places to go
Veterinary clinic
Kennel/cattery
Grooming parlour
Other people's houses
Pub/parties
School/recreation area
Fetes
Roadside
Public transport – trains, buses, etc.
Park/rural environment
Town/cities
Lifts/escalators

People and animals to meet
Men
Women
Children/babies
Elderly people
Disabled and infirm
Confident/loud people
Shy/quiet people
Delivery people – milkman, postman
People with headgear
People with glasses
People with beards
People in wheelchairs, on bicycles, pushing prams, jogging
People who differ significantly in appearance from the family members
Veterinary practice staff and others in distinctive clothing
Dogs
Other cats
Other domestic pets
Livestock

Things to encounter
Vacuum cleaners
Washing machines
Tumble dryers
Hair dryers
Vehicles
Children's toys
Pushchairs
Hot air balloons
Being alone

Activities to accept
Walking with restraint, e.g. lead or harness
Grooming/bathing
Medical examination

Table 3.3   Socialisation and habituation checklist

attention to its fear and make it worse. Owners should introduce their pet to the stimulus under controlled conditions whereby the stimulus is first presented at a considerable distance away and then gradually brought nearer. As the intensity of the stimulus is gradually increased the puppy or kitten will become desensitised to it.

The most sensitive period of development in terms of socialisation and habituation is from 4 to 14 weeks in the puppy and 2 to 7 weeks in the kitten. However, these are not rigid time limits and the process is an ongoing one (Fig. 3.3). With dogs it has been shown that under six months of age the effects of socialisation and habituation can wear off if the puppy is deprived of exposure to stimuli. This has several practical considerations:

- All puppy owners need to continually reinforce socialisation and habituation for at least the first six months.
- For puppies less than six months old, long-term stays in a kennel environment (e.g. quarantine) can be detrimental.

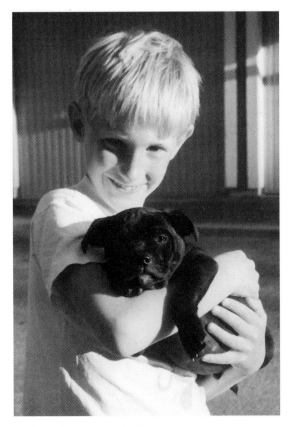

Fig. 3.3   The start of a precious new relationship.

- In situations where puppies are returned to the breeder or left at rescue societies before they are six months old it is important to realise that confinement in a kennel environment for long periods can lead to regression of socialisation and habituation.
- Puppies that are well socialised and habituated and are then moved into a different environment before six months may become unsocialised and unhabituated to the elements that are now missing, for example when moving a puppy from a city existence to a quiet rural home, or moving a puppy from a young family to a single person environment.
- The socialisation that a puppy receives from its mother and litter-mates will wear off once the puppy is placed in a new home. All puppies should therefore attend puppy playgroups in order to socialise with other dogs.

Veterinary practices can encourage owners to attend puppy parties and puppy socialisation classes or kitten information evenings in order to gain the maximum amount of information about caring for their new pet and to benefit from meeting with other new owners and their pets. These classes provide an ideal way in which to expand the practice's behavioural service and encourage a close and lasting relationship between the practice and its clients (see Chapter 9).

A list of recommended further reading for clients is given on p. 194.

Care of the Ageing Pet

4

Thomas E. Catanzaro

Pets age faster than people. This means that pets generally die within the owner's lifetime so clients have to face the ageing process and death of a pet *before* they have to face it themselves. In a society increasingly fixated on the negative aspects of ageing, this can be a frightening and difficult process.

Ageing itself is not a disease but a normal and complex biological process resulting in progressive reduction of an individual's ability to maintain homeostasis under internal physiological and external environmental stresses. This decreases the subject's viability, increases its vulnerability to disease, and eventually causes its death. Ageing is characterised by the loss of organ reserve and regenerative powers of function and adaptability.

Why should ageing be important to veterinarians? From the day we are born, we are starting to die, and the duration of life is affected by *everything* we do from the moment of birth to the time of death. The same is true for the animals in our care, which means that veterinary preventive medicine and wellness care must be a 'womb to tomb' process. In addition, veterinarians must be able to prepare the pet owner for their eventual loss. In this chapter a care programme for the ageing pet is presented, and the way to present ageing and death to pet-owners in a compassionate and caring manner is discussed.

The ageing process in pets

Most people still equate seven years of a human life to one year of a dog or cat's life although, as Table 4.1 shows, this is not actually the case.

Many factors influence the rate of ageing including breed, adult size, nutrition and life-style. Giant dog breeds such as Great Danes are generally regarded as aged by the age of five, whereas the small terriers are not geriatric until much later (Fig. 4.1). Obese animals are more at risk of dying early than those of normal weight. Purebred cats generally have a shorter life-span than mixed breeds although Siamese and Chinchillas are exceptions, with longer and shorter lives respectively. Rural cats live longer than urban cats, as do cats fed on correctly balanced commercial diets compared to those fed table scraps (Fig. 4.2).

In general it can be said that cats and dogs begin to be aged from around seven years old as it is from this age that subtle changes in organ function are first noticed. The effects of ageing are well-documented, and summarised in Table 4.2.

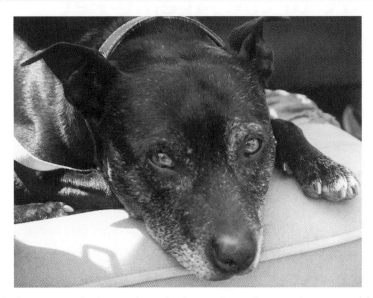

Fig. 4.1 Pets age around eight times faster than humans. Ageing changes such as greying of the muzzle and paws are typical in dogs.

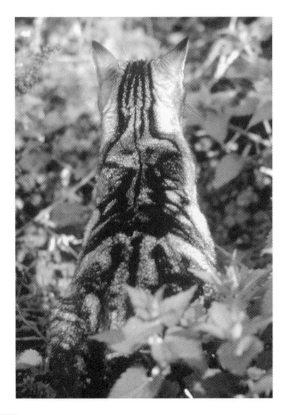

Fig. 4.2 Ageing changes in cats are often less obvious. © Ann F. Stonehouse.

Dogs do not age in the same linear fashion as people. Large breeds tend to reach maturity more slowly than small breeds, but then they age more quickly. Cats are more like small dogs. Compare the following:

Irish Terrier

Landmark	Dog	People equivalent
Sexual maturity	Birth to 6 months	Birth to mid teens
Adult muscling	6 months to 2 years	Mid teens to early 20s
Prime years	2 to 7 years	20s to early 40s
Beginning ageing	7 to 10 years	40s to 50s
Elderly	10 to 14 years	50s to 70s
Very senior	14 and above	70s and above

Saint Bernard

Landmark	Dog	People equivalent
Sexual maturity	Birth to 8 months	Birth to early teens
Adult muscling	8 months to 2.5 years	Early teens to early 20s
Prime years	2.5 to 5.5 years	20s to mid 40s
Beginning ageing	5.5 to 8 years	40s to 60s
Elderly	8 to 10 years	60s to late 70s
Very senior	10 and above	70s and above

Table 4.1 How old is your pet in 'people years'?

Ageing pets and health maintenance

The general pet population is living longer: in the United States almost half the canine and feline population are over five years old. This is the result of improved health through veterinary programmes that include vaccination, parasite control, and correct nutrition. As veterinarians give more recognition to the importance of the human–animal bond and the desire by pet-owners to prolong the healthy, active life of their old friend, there will be even more emphasis on increasing longevity and maintaining health. We are not talking about geriatric medicine – that is the science and art of taking care of *old* patients. What we are interested in is healthcare programmes that prolong youth and wellness in *middle-aged* patients.

Animals have an ability to mask disease signs; this is nature's way of assisting their survival in the wild. The clinician who waits until signs appear is into curative medicine and is already behind the power curve: elderly animals have then become 'chronic care' patients, and many require the full spectrum of alternative care programmes (homeopathy, acupuncture, chiropractic care, etc.) to maintain an adequate quality of life.

Care of the elderly pet starts at birth! The diet and preventive healthcare protection of puppies and kittens, especially during their first two years of life, affect their later years. This is not a gimmick, it is a *total healthcare plan*. However,

Ageing changes	Related clinical signs
General	
Reduced metabolism	Reduced activity
Reduced ability to thermoregulate	'Too hot in the sun, too cold in the shade'
Reduced sensitivity to thirst	Tendency towards dehydration
Changes in sleeping patterns	Frequent 'naps', irritability
Increased body fat to lean muscle ratio; loss of muscle mass	Weakness, especially in limbs
Changes in skin	Reduced elasticity
Increased sebum production	Greasy feel, smell
Changes in coat	Reduced gloss and a rough feel
Reduced grooming fastidiousness	
Decreased mental alertness	
Decreased sensitivity of senses	May become progressively blind/deaf; may lose interest in food if unable to taste it
Specific body systems	
Urinary system	Polyuria, polydipsia, incontinence, nocturia
Cardiovascular system	Signs associated with congestive heart disease
Alimentary system:	
Oral cavity	Increased incidence of calculus, and periodontal disease leading to teeth loss
Gastrointestinal	
Decreased liver function, intestinal absorption and colon motility	Reduced efficiency of digestion, flatulence, constipation
Respiratory	Obstructive lung disease, chronic bronchitis

Table 4.2 Summary of ageing changes in pets

unlike most other health programmes, despite all that you do, the pet inevitably dies. This can create problems in presenting senior healthcare both internally to staff and externally to clients, so it is important to be quite clear what the aims are for a senior wellness programme. Its aims are three-fold:

• to prevent disease by identifying and reducing risk factors;
• to identify and manage disease and age-related deterioration as early as possible to slow down further progression;

- to help the animal lead a good quality and comfortable life in its last few years.

'Quality of life' is a concept that requires discussion with the owners as definitions will vary with the individual pet, and it is an issue that will ultimately, in most cases, affect decisions concerning euthanasia. 'Quality of life' includes freedom from pain, and the ability to perform most or all normal functions such as eating, defaecating, and grooming. Depending on the animal, it may also include a variable degree of activity. For example, the owner of the aged gundog may feel the dog has reduced life quality if it can no longer follow its mistress to the shoot, or if the old cat can no longer jump up to its favourite place in the window to sun itself.

Note that there is no mention here of 'fixing' or 'curing'. The changes that are occurring are progressive and irreversible, but their *rate* of progression can be controlled in many instances.

Ageing pets are less active and have less organ reserve. Consequently, they have a decreased tolerance to the stress of nutrient excesses and deficiencies. Properly applied, a wellness programme for dogs and cats can lessen existing problems of ageing, slow or prevent pathology, and add quality years to a pet's life. Nutrition is a vital part of this process, and nutrition counselling is a service clients have come to expect from healthcare professionals.

Renal failure, for example, is among the top three causes of death in old dogs and is a primary cause of morbidity and mortality in cats. It may occur as a result of disease, ageing changes or both. Risk factors for renal failure that veterinarians should be aware of include advanced age, active renal disease, the administration of nephrotoxic drugs, concurrent disease processes, and, possibly, improper diet (Table 4.3). Dietary protein, phosphorus, and sodium excesses have all been shown to

---

Diagnostic protocol

1   Evaluate renal function regularly in older pets. Ideally, this includes yearly urinalysis and renal function tests (BUN, creatinine). This is especially important before performing invasive diagnostic or therapeutic procedures.
2   Urine specific gravity and urine protein concentrations should be monitored as a minimum. These may provide early warning indications of developing renal failure. They are also very inexpensive.
3   Monitor patients receiving nephrotoxic drugs such as some non-steroidal anti-inflammatories.

Therapeutic protocol

1   Recommend diets with restricted protein, phosphorus and sodium levels for all older pets.
2   Monitor hydration status and administer fluid therapy or diuretics as appropriate.
3   Avoid drug-induced nephrotoxicity by monitoring hydration status and drug regimes.

Table 4.3   Detecting risk factors for renal disease in ageing pets

cause or enhance the progression of renal damage. Diets that contain adequate but not excessive amounts of these nutrients slow the progression of established renal disease. They may also slow the decline in renal function that occurs with age and that may ultimately lead to renal failure. Clinical signs of decreased renal function do not occur until more than two thirds of total renal function has been lost. In addition to changes in renal function, older animals are also at risk of developing congestive heart failure and becoming obese. It is thus medically prudent to recommend diets specially designed for the nutritional needs of older animals long before clinical indications for dietary change are present.

Instigating a senior pet healthcare programme

In starting up a senior healthcare programme there are a number of important points to consider.

The value of screening

Routine screening of blood and urine is the best way to monitor the health of an older animal's major organs. Routine monitoring when the animal is healthy enables you to establish normal values. Interestingly, nearly half of clinically healthy animals will display at least one abnormal result on a 12-test serum biochemistry profile that is actually a normal result for that animal. Knowing this animal's normal values permits better interpretation of future results if the patient becomes ill.

Screening can serve a double function as a pre-anaesthetic screen. Older pets are susceptible to many of the same diseases experienced by older people such as diabetes, renal disease, heart disease, cancer and hypo- and hyperthyroidism. Disease identification *before* anaesthesia is essential to detect hidden disease and reduce the risk of post-anaesthetic complications.

Box 4.1 *Client handout 1*

The importance of blood and urine testing

In order to detect changes in organ function in the early stages, when your pet is still relatively healthy and strong, we recommend blood and urine testing as part of your pet's annual physical examination. Knowledge of the status of your pet's organ functions, hormone and electrolyte levels, and numbers of various blood cells will help us to treat your pet's problems better. The testing may also uncover further problems that we can treat before they become dangerous to your pet's health.

When your pet starts to show physical signs of ageing, we would advise twice-yearly physical examinations with follow-up blood testing as appropriate. As anaesthetics and other drugs are broken down and excreted through the liver and kidneys, if your older pet needs an anaesthetic or requires a prolonged period of drug treatment it is wise to have blood tests taken first to check organ function.

Screening helps determine whether an animal should receive a reduced dose of a medication or if the drug should be avoided altogether. For example, many common anaesthetic and analgesic drugs should be used carefully or avoided in patients with renal or hepatic insufficiency.

Owners are more willing to listen to and follow the veterinarian's advice if they understand that something is wrong. Talking through test results with an owner often results in them making diet or life-style changes for their pet (see Box 4.1).

Talking to pet-owners

Take time to talk to owners and focus on the *needs* of the ageing pet:

Mrs Powell, we all know that it is generally accepted that one year of Scruffy's life is the same as seven or eight years of our life, so by six years of age, Scruffy is ready for an 'over 40 physical', just like you!

Then explain what an 'over 40 physical' involves (see Box 4.2).

When talking to owners about problems you have identified it is important to state these clearly as needs and offer two yes options (see Box 2.1, p. 29), e.g. 'The moist sounds in Toby's chest indicate a need for chest X-rays' or 'That chronic cough (or murmur) you mentioned, Mrs Jones, indicates the need for a heart function test' or 'We need to do a full blood screen to assess Frida's excessive drinking and urinating' or 'That slow healing wound needs culture and sensitivity, and a blood test before we can decide which antibiotic is best.'

'Would you like us to start the testing today, or would you prefer to make another appointment; what would be most convenient?' Follow this with 'Once we

---

Box 4.2 Client handout 2

What is the 'over 40 physical' examination?
The 'over 40 physical' examination is a comprehensive examination of all body systems carried out at least annually to evaluate their health and function. It includes:
- history and physical examination
- routine blood profiles (biochemistry and haematology)
- endocrine evaluations as indicated
- urine analysis
- cardiopulmonary evaluation
- dental hygiene evaluation
- updating vaccination protection
- parasite prevention (internal and external)
- behaviour evaluation
- an exercise programme to keep your pet 'family fit'
- recommendations about balanced and complete nutrition suitable for the older animal

Depending on our findings we will recommend appropriate therapy and management for your pet.

have done this initial screen, there may be subsequent testing as animals often mask multiple problems and we are seeing only one sign. When I get the results, I will call you and we can talk about the findings and any sequential testing which may be necessary as our next step.'

The baseline testing offered above is not radical – it is a starting point for preventive medical care (wellness) delivery and is necessary for effective veterinary healthcare. Look at the forensic and veterinary medical logic:

The moist sounds in the thorax indicate a need for chest X-rays:

- Lesions and adhesions?
- Inhalation of foreign bodies?
- Cardiac silhouette?
- Pneumonic changes?

The chronic cough (or murmur) may indicate the need for a heart function test:

- Lead II is the initial screen; may indicate need for cardiologist referral?
- Specific valve malfunction?
- Quality and level of murmur?

The excessively urinating or drinking patient requires a full blood biochemistry and haematology screen:

- Organ malfunction?
- Absorption compromises?

The slow healing wound may need culture and sensitivity, and a blood screen:

- Biological resistance?
- Pathogen-specific chemotherapeutic regime?
- WBC response to bacterial infection?
- Atypical organisms identified?

It is important not to make the owner feel that they've done something wrong, or frighten them with words they don't really understand. 'Cancer' means death to many people: even if you qualify it by prefixing it with 'non-malignant' owners may still not fully appreciate your meaning. If they hear words they don't understand or are frightened of they stop listening. Be prepared to explain things in several different ways, and give owners plenty of chances to ask questions.

Support verbal information with written information. Various companies produce good quality client handouts that deal with the changes associated with ageing and the steps owners can take to help their pets – or you could produce your own (see Box 4.3).

Some points to bear in mind

One of the biggest problems with a wellness programme for the ageing pet is that whatever you do the animal will ultimately die: it is not a process you can stop.

Box 4.3 *Client handout 3*
Wellness care for your older pet
General introduction

Your pet is getting older, but the care you give throughout its lifetime can minimise and prevent disease as he or she ages. This wellness programme for senior pets is an example of healthcare for a life-stage. Perhaps you have already gone through our puppy/kitten care, and middle years management programmes so you will know that proper care includes periodic check-ups, routine vaccinations, parasite control, dental check-ups, regular exercise, and a good diet.

Pets age much more rapidly than humans. With the ageing process changes occur in the way the body functions. Some of these changes can be seen from the outside, for example:

- weight gain or loss;
- stiffness and difficulty going upstairs or jumping onto high surfaces;
- dull coat with an increasing amount of grey hair, especially around the muzzle;
- reduction or loss of sight or hearing.

These changes are a natural part of the ageing process and cannot be prevented, but we can help you and your pet adapt to these changes.

Advances in medicine, and better preventive care help pets live longer, healthier lives. As in human medicine, blood tests, ECGs, faecal examinations, urine analyses, and X-rays are all performed frequently on older animals because many common problems can be treated successfully if diagnosed early. Some ageing changes happen internally and can only be 'seen' by laboratory testing. In many cases, by the time your pet shows signs of illness from dysfunction of ageing organs the damage is already in the advanced stage. Many of these changes can be slowed down, and the organ function supported by correct nutrition, medication and procedures recommended by your veterinarian. With good care to promote health and prevent disease in older pets, you can help your pet remain healthy and active well into its twilight years.

One of the most important ways you can help your pet is by meeting his or her correct dietary needs. Obesity or weight loss are both common in older animals because of changes in body metabolism and activity levels. Ageing changes in the kidneys, liver and heart change a pet's requirements for sodium, phosphorus, protein and fat. Changes in the digestive processes entail an increased need for high quality nutrients and a slightly increased fibre level. Your veterinarian can help you determine the type of food that's best for your pet.

Regular examinations and follow-up care by your veterinarian will help ensure that your pet continues to be your loving companion for years to come. *Congratulations on your success in caring for your pet so well for all these years!*

This 'negative' outcome means that it is important to focus on the positive aims of ageing healthcare – to support life-long friends and companions in their last years, to help them live longer and more comfortably, and to help them maintain a good quality of life.

- The elderly animal care programmes should not be called geriatric programmes as the term 'geriatric' brings negative and rather hopeless images to mind for many clients. Healthcare for the elderly animal can be made more positive using names such as Old Friends, Golden Years, or even Elderly Care Programme.

- The 'over 40' concept is strictly an anthropomorphic introduction to the need for more care in the more senior companion animals. For instance, we promote the 'arthritis screening programme' in the autumn as a method of

---

Box 4.4 *Client handout 4*
Some practical ways you can help your older pet
General care
- Prevent access to slippery surfaces such as polished floors where animals may slip and fall.
- Set up non-slip ramps in place of steps where possible.

Feeding and digestion
- Feed an appropriate high quality, balanced commercial ration for older cats or dogs (your veterinarian can advise you).
- Raise food bowls a little above floor level to assist eating and swallowing.
- Divide the total daily ration into several smaller portions and feed more frequently.

Exercise and motion
- Encourage your pet to exercise regularly for short periods depending on its ability.
- Don't feed cats on high surfaces that they may have difficulty jumping up to.
- Lift your dog into the car or up stairs if it has trouble climbing up.

Dental care
- Pay meticulous attention to teeth and mouth with regular tooth-brushing and/or use of dental chews.

Behaviour management
- Your elderly pet may have less control of its bowels and bladder which can be distressing for both you and your pet. Ensure that your pet is not confined indoors for long periods and give it the chance to relieve itself more frequently – perhaps a friend or neighbour could help.

Poor vision and blindness
- Pets learn to cope with progressive blindness as long as big changes are not made in their environment.

Deafness
- Be extra careful with your pet near roads.

Skin and coat
- Groom regularly to help keep the coat in good condition.
- Ensure effective ecto-parasite control.

Vaccination
- To protect against life-threatening infectious diseases it is very important to keep vaccinations updated as the immune system of older animals may be less effective.

Internal parasite control
- Continue to worm regularly against internal parasites.

screening those animals that 'slow down' with the cooler weather (it is often a slower time in our clinical practice). Clients can identify with this approach to joint pain.

• The ability to start the 'Golden Years' screening with a small commitment to an initial assessment allows the client to work through their anticipatory stress, as well as the economic worries, before making the major decision.

• Chronic care of the elderly animal may require referral to an oncologist, cardiologist, or even an alternative medicine specialist. Be aware of the available professional resources and access them as you would any other specialist supporting your practice's healthcare delivery plan.

How the owner can help the aged pet

The management of the healthy older animal owes as much to the owner as to the veterinarian. There are many simple things that owners can do at home to help the pet as it ages and becomes less able. Some ideas for pet-owners are summarised in Box 4.4.

Elective euthanasia (Box 4.5)

Euthanasia is a terminal event for an animal but, if it is handled effectively, need not be a terminal experience for the client. The compassion and understanding shown during the euthanasia process, and the follow-up concern shown in bereavement

---

Box 4.5 *Euthanasia, compassion or expediency*
Pitilacker – one who is cruel to animals.
PA SPCA – new word coined 3/6/1926

Sarah, Butch, and Ralph had the same parents, but lived in different parts of the town. They met at the park most weekends and played games; they had a lot in common. They enjoyed the outdoors and the freedom to explore new worlds. In their later years, abdominal cancer beset all three ... the prognosis was poor ... each had exploratory surgery. Sarah's doctor, finding heavy metastasis, closed the abdomen, prescribed pain killers, and put Sarah in a hospice-type programme. In the case of Butch, the doctor decided that the metastasis had to be treated aggressively with chemotherapy, so he removed the major lesion and started the programme. Ralph's doctor, upon finding the metastasis, left the surgical suite, made a phone call to the family, returned to the surgical suite, and gave a lethal injection of a potent barbiturate solution.
If these doctors were licensed human physicians, two would have been paid and one would have been brought up on charges. As veterinarians, each made a legally acceptable decision; but did they make the right decision? The reason why each doctor made the decision is what determines right or wrong, not the act. The veterinary profession has the latitude to use active euthanasia as a terminal therapy; when to use this therapy is a bioethical issue, not a legal one.

mediation, can bond the client and bring them back to the practice with other animals needing a caring professional.

Animals are euthanased for various reasons which can be broadly grouped into four overlapping categories:
  1 to terminate suffering from severe injuries or serious disease;
  2 to address difficult (and unsolvable) behaviour problems;
  3 to deal with deteriorating quality of life, generally related to disease or age;
  4 for 'convenience'.

Most pet-owners instinctively know when their companion animal's battle against disease or ageing changes that affect quality of life is over. Most are also willing to concur with their veterinarian in the decision to euthanase when the situation has been honestly and clearly presented to them. However, introducing the subject of euthanasia is often not easy.

Owners are likely to have the same or similar hang-ups and worries about ageing and death as you. Some simply refuse to face the issue, finding it too painful to even think about. Your role as part of the healthcare team is to provide the professional advice that will help and support the human–animal bond through recommending what is best for the pet right to the very end. Thus, it is not appropriate to address the issue of death and dying only in the very end stages of an elderly pet's life: information about when to euthanase, burial and cremation options, and so on, should be available and even discussed with the owner long before, so that they are prepared for the event to some extent. As mentioned earlier, care of the elderly pet starts from birth: thus, a client information brochure given to the new puppy or kitten owner that contains information about the importance of health and wellness should also mention what happens at the end of a pet's life.

Understanding loss of a pet

No other medical procedure has as great an impact on you, your staff, and the quality of your veterinarian–client relationship as euthanasia. When euthanasia is performed well, it can soothe and reassure all involved that the decision to end an animal's life was correct. However, when euthanasia is performed poorly (that is thoughtlessly, or without compassion and sensitivity), it can deepen, prolong, and complicate grief for everyone.

In most family pet loss situations, the grief is severe. The pet was a member of the family and is gone. The pain felt is the price paid for the love shared, but that does not reduce the pain. Death and the loss of a loved one causes a particular sequence of behaviours and feelings first described by Dr Kubler-Ross (see Table 4.4). The loss phenomenon was later shown not to be a single sequence of feelings, but rather a cycle repeated at least four times in every stress episode (see Table 4.5). The feelings experienced during this time are a normal part of the recovery process – an important point to highlight to owners.

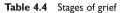

- Denial
  - Anger
    - Guilt
      - Depression
        - Acceptance

Table 4.4 Stages of grief

Anticipatory grief stage	Crisis grief stage	Crucible grief stage	Reconstructive grief stage
Anticipation	End-stage event	Immediately after	Return to senses
Emotions	*Emotions*	*Emotions*	*Emotions*
Denial with hope	Shock	Pain/fear	Sadness
Spiritual plan	Numbness	Blame/anger	New interests
Anger/guilt	Disorientation	Guilt	Self-growth
Withdrawal	Disbelief	Reminiscence	*Signs of getting stuck*
Social death rehearsal		Need to deal with emotional realities	Insomnia
Over-compensation		Develop new roles for caregivers	Weight loss/gain Increased alcoholic drinking
			Destructive behaviour

Key players:
Family Healthcare providers	Healthcare providers Significant others	Social councelors Ministry Significant others	The person himself

Adapted from: *Universal Kinship, The Bond Between All Living Things*, Latham Foundation.

Table 4.5 Loss phenomenon

A bereavement counselling service in the practice can be an invaluable way of helping clients work through their loss and come to a natural and healthy resolution. In recognition of the deep grief experienced by some owners, an increasing number of practices in the United States now offer counselling services or access to these services for owners.

In some cases, people 'get stuck' in one of the stages of grief. The practice team generally cannot be effective at this time of crisis as the client is not listening to anyone. This is the time to recommend professional counsellors such as psychologists and social workers.

The length of time it takes to work through the grief process depends on a number of factors such as the strength of the bond between owner and pet, how long they have been together, the relationship of the owner and pet (for example, was the pet the last link with a deceased child? the sole companion for a lonely, housebound person? a much-loved family member?) and the amount of external support from family and friends the grieving owner receives. In general, profound grieving for a much-loved pet can last from six months to two years before resolution is reached.

It is important that the members of a practice understand the impact of the loss phenomenon. The complex anthropomorphic relationship some people have with their animals means that loss of a pet can represent far more than loss of a close human. A pet also means different things to different family members so each individual member's reaction to illness and death must be handled differently. There are even documented cases of owners committing suicide after the death of their pets because they feel they have nothing left to live for.

Your own attitude

Working in veterinary practice you are exposed daily to other people's distress and grief. To be able to cope effectively and compassionately with this it is important to face your own fears about ageing and death. Many of us learn that it is not professional to show emotion when we euthanase animals, whatever we may be feeling inside: we do not know how to cope with a grieving owner, and are ourselves frightened at getting older and facing the prospect of eventually dying. As a result, we shy away from dealing with painful and sensitive issues such as ageing and death with our patients.★

Your attitude affects the level and success of health programmes for the ageing pet in your practice. Studies show that it is the mind-set of the healthcare provider that determines the level of care the client seeks. For example, given the three treatment modalities for cancer (medicine, surgery, euthanasia) see Box 4.5, it is the narrative of the provider, not the client, which influences the care decision (see Box 4.6).

Bioethical considerations

The application of ethics to real-life, day-to-day decision–making in healthcare delivery settings is known as bioethics. Bioethics are not clearly defined solutions

---

★ It is beyond the scope of this book to look at the issue of your own feelings during this traumatic period. Readers are preferred to the excellent book Lagoni, Butler and Hetts (1994) *The Human-Animal Bond and Grief*, for a more detailed view.

Box 4.6 *The deciding role of the veterinarian*

A study was conducted at the University of Tennessee using a double blind cast. A group of senior drama students were intensively developed as pet-owners whose family's animal companion had cancer. The second group of students were seniors in the veterinary school, and they were divided into two groups based on two pre-written scripts: one script led to euthanasia and the other led to surgery and intensive long-term care. In the final analysis, the 'veterinarian's' script decided the level of care with a 95% accuracy. This was a real-life demonstration of bioethics in action, and reflected the magnitude of the practitioner's influence.

to medical and surgical problems, rather they are the values of family, friends, colleagues, and the provider, all brought to bear upon a single healthcare situation. The healthcare alternatives in, for example, the management of malignant cancer are not based in veterinary science, they are based on personal values and practice philosophies.

The bioethics of pain and suffering

Our job as veterinarians is to prevent pain and suffering, but often we forget that they are different. Pain is physical and, in most cases, manageable with appropriate medication. Suffering has a large mental component and is much more difficult to manage. Pain often contributes to suffering, but the removal of pain does not necessarily stop suffering. For example, a dog with advancing, inoperable perianal adenomas that destroy the anal sphincter will eventually start to leak and soil the house. The dog knows that this violates the cardinal rule of the pack leader (his owners): *You do not soil the pack den.* This condition causes an anguish or suffering that we cannot directly treat in our patient. Suffering animals experience reduced quality of life and they deserve the right to euthanasia to stop the suffering, but legally animals do not have inherent rights – humans assign 'rights'. Welcome to the dilemma! (See Table 4.6.)

An interesting feature of pain and suffering prevention is that they are different, and are evaluated differently. With pain, we can do our best with the latest combinations of analgesics and can bring all our scientific skills to bear on stopping the cause of the ailment. With suffering, we have to do what is best for the patient: we must bring our ethics and feelings into the healthcare delivery setting.

To compound the problem, in preventing pain, the owner's limiting factor is generally cost. But emotions come into the critical decision process in preventing suffering. Given adequate resources, almost every pain is correctable. This cannot be said for suffering.

Patient advocacy is more than just offering the most care, or the best care: it includes offering appropriate care. As veterinary healthcare professionals, we are trained and have a responsibility to treat pain. This may be obvious to the client whose pet has just undergone surgery, but may be less obvious when an elderly

- Should a pedigreed animal with a genetic defect be eliminated from the gene pool?
- The incorrigible, vicious, unpredictable animal is a danger to human life and should be euthanased.
- The act of euthanasia is providing a humane (painless) death; but is the act kind, tender, merciful and considerate, or is it just the economic decision of a pitilacker?
- Should an abandoned animal which has become feral be eliminated?
- When an animal is a biter, chewer, digger or clawer, euthanasia is preferred over chains, kennelling or a highly restricted quality of life.
- When the economics of the family requires providing for the children *or* providing for the animal, and the animal will be replaced when the economy improves for the family, is euthanasia appropriate?
- Unwanted newborn puppies and kittens should be euthanased immediately since millions of euthanasias are performed every year in shelters and veterinary hospitals.
- An animal is legal property by law, and as such, the property owner (pet-owner) has full rights in determining the animal's disposition; veterinarians are working for the property owner, so they must abide by the society contract and meet the client's request.
- Should the veterinarian ever be the first one to mention euthanasia, or must it always be the patient's owner?
- A practice should itemise the best treatment plan, in writing with costs, then require the client to decide what they want done (or can afford to have done); neither party should be expected to compromise their position, by the other or by society.

Table 4.6   Some bioethical issues concerning euthanasia for debate

animal is presented for care. Many older animals, for example, suffer pain from dental disease to the extent of showing behavioural changes; these changes are not fully recognised by the owner until the source of pain is removed by cleaning the teeth and treating any infection (this is similar to the bitch with a grumbling pyometra whose owners comment after ovario-hysterectomy, 'She's like a new dog. We didn't realise how ill she's been all these months.').

Clients are responsible for telling us if the pain medication is not controlling the suffering (e.g. soiling the house, bumping into walls, not being able to navigate stairs, or other indicators of a deteriorating quality of life for their animal companion). This may indicate the time for euthanasia. The ability to use euthanasia methods is a privilege that we often take for granted. The debate still rages within human medical circles even though terminally ill patients may be pleading for a painless release from their suffering.

Euthanasia can be the best alternative for many reasons, of which cost may be the most obvious, but clients seldom think like this. They think about their feelings and emotions, the suffering their beloved pet may be experiencing, the decrease in the quality of life, or the pressures and demands placed on the family members who must care for the pet at home are all reasons to consider euthanasia. The feelings of each member of the family must be addressed. If we disregard the emotions of the non-paying family members, we are not much better than paid killers. If we help all the family members accept the euthanasia alternative as best for the pet, we act as facilitators of painfree death.

Conclusion

Care of the older animal is an important part of life-cycle stage health management. Slowing down the progression of age-related disease and limiting pain and suffering can give an aged pet good quality of life right up to the end. Euthanasia and death are healthcare issues that team members must help owners face up to and deal with. They must be trained to remain clear in their recommendations of what is best for the pet whilst showing compassion and understanding for the owner in their time of grief.

References and further resources

Catanzaro, T. E. (1991) *Death with Dignity, Universal Kinship, The Bond Between All Living Things*. Lathan Foundation, R&E Publications, Saratoga, California, pp. 101–118.

Lagoni, L., Butler, C. and Hetts, S. (1994). *The Human–Animal Bond and Grief*. W.B. Saunders, Philadelphia.

Macpherson, C. (1991). Setting up a geriatric healthcare programme. *Contact* (WSAVA edn), Hills Pet Products, St Albans, Herts.

Metzger, F. (1997). Help Client see geriatrics. *Veterinary Economics* **June**, 58–75.

Tilley, L.P. (1990). Nutritional risk factor management for older dogs and cats. In: *Risk Factor Management and Geriatrics*. Hills Pet Products, Lanexa, Kansas.

Wills, J. and Wolf, A. (eds) (1993). *Handbook of Feline Medicine*. Pergamon Press, Oxford.

- Delta Society (Renton, WA, 206/226–7357).
- American Animal Hospital Association: VCR three-tape series on *Pet Loss and Bereavement*. The first 45-minute tape discusses pet loss and the grief process, while the second 45-minute tape reflects on methods that the practice team can use to counsel and console clients. Each of these tapes comes with a unique workbook that is practice-specific, enabling the practice to tailor their approach to the practice philosophy. The third VCR tape in the AAHA series is sent home with the client and includes a brochure for the client to read. It is a useful aid during anticipatory grief, such as when you first discover a cancer, or when the family must move and leave the pet behind, or when congestive heart failure first becomes symptomatic. These tapes are essential for any practice that wants a team approach to client bereavement and wants to help the client to decide to return to the practice.
- *Universal Kinship, the Bond Between All Living Things*, Latham Foundation, (1991) – additional viewpoints from multiple authors about the human–animal bond.

The Role of Nutrition in Wellness Care and Obesity Management

Caroline Jevring

You are what you eat

The relationship between diet and disease in man, particularly disease of middle and old age, is a matter of public, medical and political concern, and naturally is of particular concern to the food industry. Saturated fats, sugar, salt, refined carbohydrates, vegetable fibre, additives, food hygiene, water quality and junk foods have received increasing attention over the years as having a quantifiable influence on the epidemiology of human disease.

There is also a whole art and science of nutrition for athletic performance. Top athletes eat carefully monitored amounts of essential nutrients to build and maintain ideal musculature and achieve top performance. The exact balance of nutrients varies with the level and type of training and the level of performance required.

In farm animal husbandry the importance of providing the correct nutrient balance for performance has long been appreciated. Performance here means growth and flesh production, reproduction, and milk production. In equine husbandry, horses are fed for athletic performance, and research is constantly increasing knowledge in areas such as paediatric and intensive care nutrition.

It is only relatively recently that there has been serious interest from the veterinary profession in the nutrition of companion animals. Dietary management is the lifelong, daily control of nutrient intake to meet the changing needs of a pet both in sickness and in health. Delicate changes in the pet's daily nutrient intake can have significant and profound effects on its health from affecting a life-cycle stage to damaging an organ system. Veterinarians generally accept the importance of nutritional management in disease, but apparently still lack confidence in making nutritional recommendations to maintain health, even though the provision of the correct level of nutrients for the healthy animal is as important as for the sick. Inappropriate diet is recognised as one of the major contributors to disease in exotic pets and birds. Fortunately, quality, balanced commercial diets are now available for most species.

Optimal nutritional health is an integral component and goal of wellness programmes. To best advise pet-owners and to achieve this goal, veterinarians need to know the optimal nutrient requirements of cats and dogs for dietary assessment and alteration (if necessary).

This is where the problem lies. Up until the last few years, clinical nutrition of companion animals, especially nutrition of the healthy animal, was taught only at the most rudimentary level at veterinary colleges. Veterinarians qualified knowing everything about feeding cattle and pigs, but precious little about the correct nutrition of pets – a weakness hungrily seized upon by commercial petfood companies. Through vigorous advertising they persuaded pet-owners that their products were the best for their pets. The results are impressive: in Britain, owners of the 6.5 million dogs and 7 million cats spend billions of pounds annually on petfoods and associated products.

Then the companies realised they could go a stage further and produce diets with a veterinary seal of approval. The best of these companies mounted massive education campaigns for veterinary surgeons and their staff, teaching them about nutrition of healthy and sick animals, and how to market and sell the products the company manufactured. Armed at last with this knowledge and with top quality products from serious, committed manufacturers, veterinarians could now talk confidently about dietary management of both sick and healthy pets. But whereas they could justify recommendations about the nutritional needs of sick pets, in accordance with the tradition that a veterinary practice is a place to treat the sick, they still stumbled over talking convincingly to owners about the nutritional requirements for maintenance of health.

In the 1980s the world economy crashed. In order to survive, companion animal practitioners were forced to look seriously at the true needs of their market – pet-owners and their pets. They realised that owners wanted optimal healthcare for their pets, including nutritional advice, and marketing petfood for healthy pets suddenly became attractive. But by now veterinarians faced huge problems from their clients: the veterinary practice was not the place to buy petfood! What were these premium quality, limited retail outlet petfoods anyway – just an expensive way to fleece the client?

Fortunately, veterinarians have persisted and caring clients realise that the veterinarian really is the best authority on what is right for their pet to keep it healthy through its different life-stages. They acknowledge that the premium quality diets veterinarians recommend and, in many cases, sell really do make a difference to their pet's health. They appreciate that their veterinarian has reviewed the vast array of petfoods on the market and, using his professional knowledge, selected only the best.

Marketing nutrition to pet-owners

For veterinarians to effectively market premium nutritional products to their clients they need first to understand how people buy petfoods (see Table 5.1). The most important factors that influence owners are that the pet likes the food, the price is right, and the apparent contents. Owners, in fact, tend to buy from a mixture of emotional and garbled 'fact' reasons: 'apparent contents', for example, means the presence of meat/fish for dogs/cats respectively because everyone 'knows' dogs/cats *need* meat/fish.

My pet likes variety.	Based on human values, petfood manufacturers encourage this demand for flavours as they sell more product. Often the basic ingredients in the different varieties are the same: flavour is altered using 'digest', a breakdown product from decomposed animal and vegetable matter. There is no evidence that animals *need* or seek flavour variety although they can become *accustomed* to it.
It's easiest to buy the petfood at the supermarket when I do the weekly shopping, and they have such a good choice.	Commercial companies have cashed in on selling through convenience outlets. For some owners it may require quite an effort to make a separate journey to the veterinarians.
A cheap petfood'll do for my pet. **or** *I always get those expensive luxury foods for my pet – she deserves only the best.*	20% of purchases are made primarily on price – at both ends of the range. Owners in this category either perceive petfood as something to feed the pet that keeps it alive, or as a symbol of the owners love and devotion.
I've always fed …	Both brand loyalty (defined as a repeated action that becomes a habit) and traditional feeding methods influence choice.
Cats need fish. Dogs need meat.	Popular misconceptions: some animals prefer fish/meat but dogs, for example, are omnivores and can even thrive on a balanced vegetarian diet.
I always prepare his food myself.	Some owners still prefer to prepare their pet's food from scratch, believing this must be best. Such diets run the risk of being severely unbalanced because of the cooking process.
He likes those meaty chunks.	Product appearance is more important to owners than to their pets. Gourmet products may appear to contain a substantial amount of skeletal muscle (meat) but actually contain a variety of animal by-products and textured vegetable protein (TVP), which is composed of extruded soy flour mixed with red or brown colouring to make it resemble chunks of meat or liver.
It's important his bowels move well every day.	So-called evidence of 'healthy bowels' is actually the product of low-digestibility ingredients. Large volumes of stool are not a necessary component of good health.
I like to see her eat well	Feeding is often equated with giving love. Feeding lots means giving lots of love to the pet. This can be achieved through feeding low-quality, low-digestibility pet foods (the animal is foced to eat large quantities to get the nutrients it needs) and/or overfeeding.
We need to cut down her calorie intake a bit.	'Low-calorie' petfoods follow the human fad for these products associated with a healthier approach to eating. On analysis, many turn out to have the same or even higher calorie levels on a dry matter basis than ordinary petfoods.

Table 5.1 Why people buy petfoods

By understanding what influences client purchases the veterinarian can selectively use the same arguments to sell the products he recommends. The difference is that in buying from the veterinarian, owners are assured of premium products of the highest quality that are suited to the animal's life-cycle stage and selected according to the veterinarian's knowledge and understanding of the animal's nutritional needs.

Average pet-owners know little about their animal's nutritional needs and are thus quite susceptible to skillfully presented advertising claims, whether or not the claims are valid. Many marketing organisations use a variety of these claims so that if one does not appeal to a particular owner, perhaps another will (see Table 5.2).

'Fresh' ingredients	As opposed to stale?
Addition/removal of special ingredients – the the magic × ingredient that cures all problems – or causes them.	Pet-owners seek products with (real) meat/without meat, with added vitamins/without vitamin E, and so on. Most of these are fads based on ignorance and manipulation by the popular press.
'New' flavours	Increases the range of choice, and therefore the sales. Some combinations are quite extraordinary.
Canned versus dried food	Canned food is often perceived as being 'nicer' than dried. British culture is still heavily influenced by the 'meat (canned animal by-products) and biscuit' philosophy for feeding dogs. However, complete dried rations are becoming more popular as convenience foods. Cat owners are concerned about the relationship of dry diet to bladder disease.
Packaging size	Packaging needs to range from 'convenience' for the person needing small quantities to 'economy' for those with five large dogs.
Price	20% of people select products primarily on price (see above).
Guilt: *If you love your pet you'll feed it xyz. Give your pet what you know s/he loves … Your friend deserves only the best. Feed …*	Television advertising in particular uses guilt to manipulate people to buy for their pets, playing on themes such as reward of devoted love, luxury treats for your faithful friend, and so on.
Professional recommendations – usually from breeders	Breeders provide the first contact with new owners and can be remarkably influential in their recommendations. The theory is that successful breeders should know what is best for their animals.

Table 5.2 Some ways in which petfood companies influence petfood purchases

Talking facts

The veterinarian is the only person qualified to give the facts about optimal nutrition, but owners will seldom take up recommendations presented as pure fact. Veterinarians and their staff need to be able to talk about palatability, price and daily feeding costs, the advantages of balanced complete foods, the significance of certain nutrients on a pet's health and so on, in terms that the owner can understand. For example, telling a cat owner that a particular premium diet has so many mg/kg of magnesium is probably meaningless to the owner, whereas explaining that this diet is low in the mineral magnesium, which reduces the chances of the cat developing bladder stones, is far more understandable.

The veterinarian's attitude

Should veterinarians recommend and sell petfoods for healthy pets? Yes! There are many reasons:

- Animals go through several critical life-stages between birth and death when physiological changes alter the need for and sensitivity to certain nutrients. For example, a pet's requirement for calcium is higher during growth and lactation than during normal adult maintenance; phosphorus, sodium and protein intake should be reduced in the diet of older animals to help support function in ageing organs.
- Some animals are prone to diseases whose onset and progression may be nutritionally influenced. The veterinarian's role is to identify these at-risk animals and make especially sure that owners are aware of the nutritional factors that may affect their health. Cavalier King Charles Spaniels, for example, have a hereditary tendency to develop early congestive heart failure associated with valve degeneration. Many commercial petfoods contain unnecessarily high levels of sodium. By feeding a low salt diet throughout the pet's life the onset of clinical illness may be delayed. Neutered cats are predisposed to formation of bladder struvite and obesity, both of which may be controlled by feeding a low magnesium, acid urine forming, calorie-restricted food. Skeletal disease in large breed puppies due to overnutrition can be prevented by feeding carefully regulated quantities of a balanced diet for growth.
- It is no longer adequate for veterinarians to rely on recommending a 'popular brand' when owners request information about correct nutrition. There is such a vast array of diets to choose from that pet-owners can feel quite overwhelmed; they then select a food based on advertising claims, breeder recommendations, or the advice of a friend – reasons which we have already seen are not in the best interests of the animal. Sceptical veterinarians should compare for themselves the perceptible difference in animal health of those fed on 'ordinary' or premium quality petfood. The author's own 'Aha!' experience with nutrition for the healthy pet came from seeing the visible health and activity differences apparent in old dogs converted onto a

premium quality senior diet. Within the space of a few weeks, dogs that had been generally 'aged' in their attitude and behaviour show a whole new lease of life. Owners report that their old pets can jump in and out of the car again, jump fences, and climb stairs, coat quality and appearance improves, and their pets show a new interest in life.

- Nutrition is profitable. It is only a short step for veterinarians to go from recommending premium healthcare products to selling them. It is made more profitable by the fact that much of the advisory counselling can be done by trained support staff, and there are some excellent training programmes available from leading petfood manufacturing companies.

Dietary management and wellness

Advising pet-owners about optimal nutrition is integral to all wellness programmes. The actual needs in each programme are presented in the relevant chapters but the following description of managing obesity highlights some of the problems associated with talking to owners. The feeding of pets is made very complex by the intricacies of the human–animal bond. It is the veterinarian's obligation to present the facts and ensure that owners have the best possible chance to provide optimal nutrition for their pet.

An approach to the management of the obese pet in veterinary practice

Obesity is the most common disease of malnutrition, affecting 10–40% of pets (Mason, 1970; Edney and Smith, 1984; Hand et al, 1989; Bush, 1993). It is defined as a complex, treatable, clinical syndrome of multifactorial origin with multiple interlinked sequelae (Table 5.3); however, the basic problem is that the animal eats more calories than it needs. The detrimental effects of obesity are well documented (Crane, 1991) although fortunately many of them of them are reversible when the

---

- Breed
- Age
- Sex
- Neutering
- Lack of exercise
- Feeding highly palatable foods (e.g. many supermarket brands, table scraps, food for human consumption)
- Inappropriate feeding habits (e.g. giving treats, table scraps, etc.)

Table 5.3 Predisposing factors for obesity

- Hormone-related disorders (e.g. diabetes mellitus, altered metabolism)
- Degenerative and traumatic arthroses
- Cardiovascular changes (e.g. hypertension, increased airway resistance)
- Dermatological disorders (e.g. lipomas, skin-fold dermatoses)
- Reduced exercise tolerance
- Reduced life quality
- Increased surgical risk

In cats there is a predisposition to hepatic lipidosis.

In humans there is reduced life expectancy and increased risk of serious infection.

Table 5.4 Detrimental effects of obesity

patient returns to or approaches ideal weight (Table 5.4). Obesity is one of the most challenging conditions for veterinary surgeons to manage effectively. This is not because slimming an overweight pet is difficult, but because success depends completely on gaining the cooperation of the pet-owner, who is often fundamental to both the cause and the treatment of the condition.

One of the long-term aims of an obesity programme is to teach owners to recognise obesity and its inherent risks, and to take responsibility for managing the problem. They are rewarded with a happier, healthier, and more enjoyable companion.

The following explains how to set up an effective weight management programme in practice, and highlights the importance of gaining owner cooperation at every step of the way. The desire to over-feed a pet to the point of obesity is based on a key component of the human–animal bond: the giving and receiving of 'love'. The owner gives the pet who is always begging ('hungry') extra food and treats ('love') that the pet relishes and, in return, receives their pet's devoted and affectionate companionship.

Many owners don't want to diet their overweight pet because:
- they think it is 'cruel';
- they are afraid the pet will reject and hate them;
- they have been unsuccessful with diets themselves;
- they don't understand the seriousness of the health risks associated with obesity;
- they think a single diet food is boring;
- changing feeding habits is inconvenient.

Raising client awareness of obesity as a problem

Many owners do not understand the health risks associated with obesity, so the veterinary practice needs to raise their awareness, starting from the first visit to the clinic with a new puppy or kitten. This is especially important with the obesity-prone breeds such as Labradors.

Methods that can be used in the clinic (Macpherson, 1992) include:

- Weigh and record the pet's weight on every visit to the clinic so that clients see that weight is an important indicator of health.
- Weigh all pets routinely, not just the overweight ones, so that the owners of obese animals don't feel picked on.
- Discuss correct nutrition with owners on a regular basis to encourage them to feed their pets correctly, and to ask the veterinary surgeon for advice.
- Place walk-on platform scales and weight charts in the reception area, and have a trained member of staff available to help weigh the pets. Weight is an important health parameter, and owners can immediately see that their pet is overweight if they can compare their pet's weight with the ideal breed weight.
- Be able to discuss why obesity is a health risk to the pet, because owners don't appreciate that obesity can be a life-threatening condition.
- Be prepared to discuss owners' fears about dieting.
- Discuss inappropriate feeding habits such as giving treats, titbits and table scraps.
- Discuss risk factors for obesity and how they can be managed.

PREVENTION IS BETTER THAN CURE

Owners often do not perceive their overweight pet as being at risk because:
- 'fat is happy';
- they are often overweight themselves;
- they don't understand the health risks;
- weight gain happens insidiously so they often don't realise their pet is overweight;
- being overweight is 'normal' for the breed, e.g. show Labradors, Pugs;
- they are proud of their pet's size and find it comical.

Identifying obesity

An obese pet is defined as being 15% or more over its ideal weight (Lewis, 1987). This may be only 330 g for a Chihuahua but over 7.5 kg for a Rottweiler. Fat is laid down slowly and insidiously, so owners often don't realise how overweight their pet has become. They rarely, if ever, visit the practice to ask for help with their pet's weight problem – they come because their pet has some other problem, which may, in fact, be due to the obesity.

Weighing on easy-to-use, walk-on platform scales and comparing the weight with an optimal breed weight chart is the easiest method to identify obesity and is one with which owners are familiar. Another simple, but less accurate, method is to feel gently over the ribcage to assess the fat layer under the skin. You should be able to feel the ribs as your hands spread over the ribcage.

Other methods, such as taking girth and height measurements and calculating the expected weight, or weighing by subtraction on bathroom scales, are complicated, inaccurate and lead to confusion.

It is important that the veterinary surgeon confirms the diagnosis of obesity during a clinical examination to eliminate possible confusion with, say, pregnancy or ascites.

It is important to use an appropriate term when speaking to owners about their overweight pet. Using the word 'obesity' can conjure up terrible visions of grossly overweight pets which many owners may not be able to identify with. 'Overweight' is much better than 'fat', but 'tubby' and 'cuddly' may detract from the seriousness of the problem.

Starting on a weight management programme

There are several ways to slim a pet but some methods are better and more effective than others. Weight loss in pets is achieved by client co-operation to reduce the calorie intake and increase the rate of calorie usage through exercise.

The role of the family

Commitment by the owner and their family to a weight loss programme for their pet is essential for success. By having some background information on the family and the pet's diet history, and by involving the whole family from the beginning, obstacles to success can be anticipated and solutions found for them.

Questions to ask the family include:
- Who feeds the pet and when?
- What foods is the pet given?
- How much is fed daily, including titbits?
- How often is the pet fed?

The long-term aim is to educate clients about optimal health for their pet through good eating habits. Many pet owners are overweight themselves. To reduce embarrassment when talking to them about the problems of obesity, link anything you say to their pet and their pet's health.

The role of diet

An animal becomes overweight because it eats more calories than it requires for normal maintenance. Thus, to reduce its weight, the pet's calorie intake must be decreased to the point where the pet is actually using its body stores of calories, i.e. its fat. As the aim is to achieve slow, steady weight loss, calorie restriction should be around 40% (dogs) and 25% (cats) of the requirement for *maintenance of ideal weight* (Lewis, 1987). The animal may need to be calorie-restricted for several months to achieve the desired weight loss, so it is important that it is fed a balanced and nutritionally complete calorie-restricted diet. Using an unbalanced diet in this situation may produce a dangerous deficiency state (Van Itallie and Young, 1984).

One of the advantages of changing on to a new food when the pet 'goes on a diet' is to make the owner change feeding habits and accept that the pet really is on a special food for its weight problem.

Owners often claim that the volume of food they give their overweight pet is small. In fact, as an overweight animal needs fewer calories to maintain its fat weight than when it is a normal weight, this may genuinely be true. However, many owners do not perceive that the constant little snacks they give their pet throughout the day PLUS this small volume of food adds up to more calories than the animal needs.

The role of exercise

A slow and careful increase in the amount of daily exercise helps to burn off excess calories and improve general condition.

Choice of diet for weight loss

Commercial low-calorie diets

There are several different types of commercial weight-reducing diet available to veterinary surgeons. Basically these can be divided into three groups: very high fibre, moderate fibre, and low fibre.

- *Very high fibre*. Using a low fat, high fibre (more than 15% dry matter) diet that is nutritionally complete and balanced has repeatedly proven to be the most effective method available for weight loss (Lewis, 1987; Hand, 1988). The role of fibre in weight loss is summarized in Table 5.5 but, in addition, a high fibre diet is of benefit in managing certain obesity-related conditions such as diabetes mellitus. The calorie reduction, around 40% compared to a normal maintenance diet, and the high fibre content mean that only the calorie intake, not the volume of food the pet receives, is reduced – an important factor in owner co-operation for those owners who perceive dieting ('cutting back') to be unkind.
- *Moderate fibre diets*. The physiological effects of the fibre are much less significant in the moderate fibre diets (around 7% DM). Calorie reduction is achieved through replacing some dietary fat, a concentrated form of calories, with less calorie-dense carbohydrate. It is less easy to produce satiety at the same level of calorie restriction that is achieved with the high fibre diets. With no fixed formula, and less regulation of nutrient levels, these diets are also less suitable for longer-term weight loss, especially in older pets and pets with obesity-related conditions.

> 15% fibre on a dry matter basis causes:

- satiety, with a low fat diet
- 'dilution' of calories
- decreased rate of digestion
- reduced nutrient assimilation
- slowed transit time through the small intestine.

It also aids in the management of secondary diabetes mellitus.

Table 5.5 The role of fibre in weight management

- *Low fibre diets.* These contain the levels of fibre found in ordinary petfoods (around 2–3%), so can claim no consistent satiety effect at all. Water is rapidly absorbed from the stomach and small intestine, does not slow gastric emptying, fails to provide a sustained feeling of gastrointestinal fullness, and does not reduce energy nutrient digestibility and assimilation. Many of these diets have an energy density similar to regular maintenance diets on a dry matter basis, and, in effect, are equivalent to feeding less of a regular petfood.

'Light' products

The term 'light' to imply lower in calories has become commercially acceptable in both human and animal products. However, the term is meaningless and some popular supermarket brands of petfood with a 'light' label have the same calorie density on a dry matter basis as ordinary supermarket brands.

Misleading label descriptions on certain 'light' brands imply that they can be used to reduce weight. However, 'light' products are not suitable for weight loss as they are not sufficiently calorie restricted. Some of the reputable premium brands of 'light' products, which are genuinely calorie-restricted and are not available in supermarkets, can be used for prevention of weight gain and in long-term weight management.

Adding fibre in the form of vegetables and/or bran

Vegetables have a relatively low insoluble fibre:wet volume ratio, and wheat bran is only 12.5% fibre DM, so very large quantities of either/both would be needed to significantly raise the fibre content of an ordinary petfood. At the levels required it would be impossible to maintain palatability, and nutrient availability would be severely compromised.

Recipes for vegetable-based, low-calorie, weight-losing diets exist, but ensuring that they are balanced for long-term use, and maintaining client co-operation in preparing and using them may be difficult.

Reducing the amount of food currently fed

To achieve weight loss through calorie reduction, the amount of a pet's *regular* food needs to be reduced by 30% (cat) to 40% (dog). This method does not usually work well at home because the pet:

- is often hungry;
- is more inclined to beg for food;
- may suffer nutrient deficiencies if it is on a reduced ration for a prolonged period.

In addition it does not represent a significant change in the feeding habits and therefore is not easy for the owner to maintain.

Changing the ratio of canned food to biscuit

Altering the ratio of food types has little significant effect on the intake of calories.

Starvation

Confining an animal and giving it no food and only water will cause it to lose weight, but is neither humane nor effective in the long term. Obese cats treated in this manner are predisposed to hepatic lipidosis, which may be fatal. There are a few known health detriments to dogs (such as changes in the gut), and there are a number of disadvantages:

- Weight loss is only slightly faster than with moderate calorie restriction.
- Total calorie restriction is expensive as it requires hospitalisation.
- This method is not based on gaining owner co-operation and understanding, so owners will revert to old habits when the pet returns home.

Quantity to feed

If using a commercial weight-reducing diet, follow the feeding guides provided by the manufacturer, based on the ideal weight of the pet. This quantity should be divided into several smaller amounts to help keep the animal feeling satiated and increase meal-induced heat loss. If there is a less than 10% weight loss from the starting weight after four weeks then consider reducing the amount fed (but see *Problems with weight loss*).

Regardless of the diet used, the client must follow instructions explicitly and feed only the specific amount of food prescribed.

Calculating the ideal weight

Ideal weight can be estimated from breed weight charts, and approximations made for mongrels. Normal weights for cats are not well documented and range from 2–7 kg depending on the basic size of the cat. These weights are only guides and there must be allowances for individuals. Thus, the final weight of the pet may be different from the calculated weight if it suits the animal better, as the 'ideal' weight is only an estimate of normality.

If the animal is grossly overweight it may be easier for the owner to achieve the weight loss by breaking up the amount to be shed into smaller portions, e.g. a 65 kg Rottweiler might need to lose 25 kg: this could be broken up into goals of 5 kg units each.

How long will it take to reach the ideal weight?

It is important for owners to appreciate that weight loss is not achieved overnight. To give them an approximate idea of how long their pet will need to be on a calorie-reduced diet, the time needed to reach the ideal weight can be roughly calculated based on the expected weekly rate of weight loss:

- up to 0.25 kg for a cat or small breed of dog;
- 0.25–0.5 kg for a medium sized dog;
- 0.5–1 kg for a large breed.

The weekly weight loss divided into the total required weight loss provides the period required to achieve that weight loss.

Monitoring progress

One of the most important parts of a successful weight loss programme is to monitor the progress of the patient on a frequent and regular basis. Ideally, this is at 2-week intervals: long enough for the pet to have lost measurable weight, but short enough for the owner to keep the commitment. Marking the weight on a chart for the owners allows them to follow the progress of their pet easily.

Regular monitoring also helps overcome crises the owner might have, such as when a relative comes to stay who feeds the dog titbits (Table 5.6), or when the dog raids the dustbin. Encouraging support can really spur owners on, especially as they begin to see and experience the difference in their pets.

Problems with weight loss

Sometimes the animal does not lose the expected amount of weight. If this occurs over two or more weighings then a detailed investigation should be carried out

The feeding of titbits and treats is contraindicated for several reasons:

- they contribute excess calories
- they predispose to obesity
- they encourage begging
- they are part of a poor feeding pattern.

However, giving a treat is a very special interaction for some owners. Rather than ban treats altogether and have the owner not comply with the diet regime, it is better to allow a certain number of treats *but* by replacing a portion of the measured daily allowance of diet food by the treat. By doing this, you show that you recognise the importance of this interaction for the owner, but at the same time highlight the importance of the pet being on a strictly controlled diet.

Table 5.6 Titbits and treats

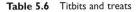

into how the owner is feeding the pet. The most common reasons for the pet not to lose weight are:

- it is receiving additional food, i.e. the owner is feeding more of the diet food and/or other food as well, or the pet is scavenging,
- the initial calorie restriction is not sufficient; in this case the quantity of diet food needs to be recalculated.

Giving the owner a chart to fill in of everything that the pet consumes over 24 hours may reveal the source of the problem, otherwise hospitalisation may be necessary to ensure restriction of the calorie intake. In a small percentage of failure cases, undiagnosed disease such as hypothyroidism may be the cause of the problem.

Achieving target weight

Achieving target weight is only part of the battle against obesity. An animal that has been overweight is prone to become overweight again. To help prevent this, the pet should be maintained on a calorie-restricted, low fat, high fibre diet, and regularly weighed. High quality prescription-type and light diets are suitable in this situation. The daily ration should be divided into at least two portions to help maintain a feeling of satiety, and the pet re-weighed every two to three months.

Other options such as putting the pet back on to its old food or on to a premium quality, calorie-dense maintenance diet, are generally unsatisfactory and tend to predispose to weight gain.

Who is responsible for running the obesity programme?

For maximum effectiveness, everyone in the practice should accept a weight management programme and agree a protocol for it, even though there may only be a few people directly involved with it on a daily basis.

Although a veterinarian must make the diagnosis of obesity, this programme is ideal for suitably trained vet nurses to run. One of their key roles is in establishing a strong client bond, which gives both job and personal satisfaction. Training and advice on setting up programmes are available from petfood manufacturing companies.

When do we run it?

Programmes are run in different ways in different practices. Successful arrangements for clients include:

- individual appointments with a specialised nurse during normal surgery hours;
- having a group meeting of dieting patients run by a trained nurse at a quiet time of the day, or after surgery hours;
- appointments between certain times of day and/or on certain days to see the nurse.

The more flexibility that the client has for making appointments the greater the chance of co-operation with the programme.

Marketing your programme

Taking every opportunity to talk about the problems of obesity, and making weighing part of every clinical examination are the two most important ways of marketing your programme.

Displays in the reception area of posters, dietary products, before and after photos, information leaflets, weighing scales, weight charts and so on, catch the clients' eyes as they walk in.

Newsletters, client brochures and targeted mailings can contain information about the new service. In addition, your programme can be externally marketed through meetings at local breeder clubs, articles in the local paper, or on local radio and TV.

Looking at the costs involved

The major cost of setting up a good obesity programme is the purchase of walk-on, platform scales, but this can be rapidly offset by profits from increased sales of dietary products. The petfood companies that manufacture the dietary foods produce good client information brochures, weight charts and posters as a service to their customers so it is not necessary to produce your own.

Practices can also create an income from charging for the programme in different ways:

- charge for the initial veterinary consultation and all subsequent nurse consultations,
- charge for the initial vet consultation followed by free nurse consultations,
- charge a fee for going on the programme, part of which may be redeemed when the ideal weight is reached,
- as above, plus 'fining' the client a small amount and giving the money to a charity if the pet does not lose weight.

The profit, which can be substantial, comes primarily from the sales of dietary foods, and the increased opportunities for other business from the clients.

Measuring the programme's success

No programme should ever be set up in a practice without the means to measure its success. Factors that can be measured include:
- the number of clients that take up the programme compared to the anticipated number;
- the number of pets that successfully reach target weight;
- the increased level of owner awareness of pet obesity;
- the increased income from sales of diets.

Conclusion

With planning and organisation, setting up and running a weight management programme in your practice is fun and rewarding. The practice benefits from having an obesity programme through raising awareness of a common disease problem, improving the health, life quality and life expectancy of the pets in its care, and increasing the enjoyment the owner can have from a happier, livelier pet.

References

Anderson, R.S. (1990). Nutrition in practice – why bother? *Journal of Small Animal Practice* **31**, 473–476.

Bush, B.M. (1993). Obesity in small animals, its causes, diagnosis and treatment. *Veterinary Practice Clinical Review* **1**(6), 1–2, 4, 6–7.

Crane, S.W. (1991) Occurrence and management of obesity in companion animals. *Journal of Small Animal Practice* **32**, 275–282.

Earle, K.E. (1990). Feeding for health. *Journal of Small Animal Practice* **31**, 477–481.

Edney, A.T.B. and Smith, P.M. (1986). Study of obesity in dogs visiting veterinary practices in the UK. *Veterinary Record* **118**, 391–396.

Hand, M.S. (1988). Treating and preventing obesity in small animals. In: *Managing Fibre Responsive Diseases*. Veterinary Medical Publishing Company, Lenexa, p 28–35.

Hand, M.S., Armstrong, P.J. and Aller, T.A. (1989). Obesity: occurrence, treatment and prevention. *Veterinary Clinics of North America* **19**(3), 447–474.

Lewis, L.D. (1987). *Obesity: a Commentary on Nutritional Management of Small Animals*. Mark Morris Associates, Topeka, Kansas, p 1–34.

Lewis, L.D. Morris, M.L. and Hand, M.S. (1987). *Small Animal Clinical Nutrition*. Mark Morris Associates, Topeka, Kansas.

Macpherson, C. (1992). Ten points to help owners recognize obesity. *Progress through Partnership* **Autumn**, Hills Pet Products, UK.

Mason, E. (1970). Obesity in pet dogs. *Veterinary Record* **86**, 612.

Van Itallie, T.B. and Yang, M.U. (1984). Cardiac dysfunction in obese dieters: a potentially lethal complication of rapid, massive weight loss. *American Journal of Clinical Nutrition* **39**, 695–702.

Management of Dental Disease

6

Cecilia Gorrell

Our dogs and cats suffer from similar diseases of the oral cavity as we do. Of the conditions seen in a small animal practice, periodontal disease is the most common. The great majority of dogs and cats over the age of three years have a degree of periodontal disease which warrants intervention (Gorrell and Robinson, 1995).

Periodontal disease is a collective term for a number of inflammatory conditions affecting the periodontium or supporting apparatus of the tooth. The primary cause of periodontal disease is the presence of plaque on the tooth surfaces. Dental plaque is composed of aggregates of bacteria and their by-products, salivary components, oral debris, and occasional epithelial and inflammatory cells. It accumulates rapidly on a clean tooth surface. Undisturbed plaque will cause a marginal gingivitis within four to five weeks (Lindhe et al, 1975). Gingivitis is the initial lesion of periodontal disease. In a proportion of individuals, untreated gingivitis will progress to periodontitis with destruction of the periodontal ligament and alveolar bone. The end result of periodontitis is the loss of an otherwise healthy tooth.

There is good circumstantial evidence that a focus of infection in the mouth in individuals with periodontitis may induce disease at distant sites, e.g. kidneys and heart valves, as a result of bacteraemic spread (DeBowes et al, 1996). Moreover, periodontitis may well cause discomfort to the affected animal. Consequently, the maintainance of a healthy oral cavity is of importance for the general health and welfare of the dog and cat.

Aetiology and pathogenesis of periodontal disease

It used to be thought that all individuals were susceptible to periodontitis and thus that all cases of gingivitis progressed to periodontitis with consequent bone loss and eventual tooth loss. It was also accepted that the susceptibility to periodontitis increased with increasing age. We now know that it is only some individuals with gingivitis that progress to periodontitis. Also, it is often only at certain sites in the oral cavity where disease progresses. Periodontitis is now seen as resulting from a complex interplay of bacterial infection and host response, modified by behavioural factors (Slots and Taubman, 1992; Lindhe, 1993; Loe and Brown, 1993; American Academy of Periodontology, 1996; Revert et al, 1996; Lange et al 1997).

Tissue-destructive periodontal diseases can be considered as a series of infections, affecting single or multiple sites in the oral cavity. All affected sites within an individual do not seem to express disease activity, i.e. are not actively progressive, at all times.

Data from several studies indicate that certain micro-organisms should be considered as periodontal pathogens or as a periodontitis-associated microflora. However, the number of bacteria must exceed a certain threshold level in order to induce disease activity. Thus, the mere presence of a certain periodontal pathogen does not necessarily indicate that the individual will develop periodontal disease.

It thus appears that the development of periodontal disease is dependent on the simultaneous presence of multiple factors:

- The host must be susceptible for disease progression, both locally and systemically.
- The local environment must contain micro-organisms that reinforce the infection, or at least do not prevent the disease-evoking activity.
- The local environment must allow for pathogenic factors to be expressed by the micro-organism.
- The pathogen has to be present in sufficient numbers to be able to induce disease progression.

Fortunately it is not common for all these factors to be present at the same time.

Factors which predispose to plaque accumulation

Factors which predispose to plaque accumulation should be removed. Such factors include:

- overcrowding of teeth, e.g. brachycephalic breeds and small dogs;
- other malocclusions;
- retained deciduous teeth;
- fractured teeth, as exposed dentine provides a roughened surface.

Situations when oral defences are compromised

In the management of periodontal disease it is essential to ensure that the animal is otherwise healthy. Any concurrent disease needs identification and appropriate treatment. In situations where the individual's ability to mount an inflammatory reaction in response to trauma is diminished, more intensive oral hygiene requirements are needed to maintain periodontal health. Situations when oral defences may be compromised include:

- reduced production/flow of saliva;
- immunosuppression;
- renal failure;
- malnutrition;

- stress;
- other systemic diseases.

Systemic complications of periodontal disease

It should always be remembered that a focus of infection in the oral cavity such as severe periodontitis can act as a reservoir of infection for the whole body. Bacteria enter the bloodstream via inflamed gums. These bacteria may settle in other organs, e.g. kidneys, liver, heart, or possibly lungs, and interfere with the function of these organs.

Diagnosis of periodontal disease

A full examination of the oral cavity is only possible with the animal under general anaesthesia. However, a lot of information can be gained from a conscious examination. Most animals will allow you to lift the lip and pull back the cheek to expose the buccal surfaces of the teeth and the gingiva. If handled gently but firmly, most animals will also let you open the mouth to get a quick view of the occlusal tooth surfaces as well as the lingual and palatal aspects.

Conscious examination

Gingivitis manifests as a red and swollen gingival margin which is prone to bleeding on manipulation, e.g. on brushing. In severe cases, gingival haemorrhage is spontaneous.

Gingival recession and furcation exposure are indicative of breakdown of the periodontium and are signs of periodontitis. Purulent discharge from the gingival sulcus and tooth mobility also indicate progressive and usually severe periodontitis.

Examination under general anaesthesia

A complete examination of the oral cavity involves mucous membranes, tongue and pharynx as well as the teeth and their supporting apparatus. Intraoral radiography is an important part of a full clinical examination. Without radiographs the bone and periodontal ligament are not visualised and assessment of attachment loss is not possible.

Periodontitis is diagnosed based on probing sulcus depth using a blunt periodontal probe. A sulcus depth in excess of 3 mm is usually indicative of breakdown of the periodontal ligament and alveolar bone and is considered a pathological pocket. Pocket depth is not an accurate method of recording tissue destruction as the concurrent presence of gingival oedema or hyperplasia will yield a false pocket depth. A more accurate way of measuring loss of attachment is to measure from a known point on the tooth, usually the cemento–enamel junction, to the base of the sulcus or pocket. Loss of alveolar bone is diagnosed radiographically. From a treatment point of view it is important to differentiate between horizontal and vertical bone loss in periodontitis as the treatment will differ.

All findings should be recorded to allow treatment planning. There are several charts available on the market or you could make your own. Fig. 6.1 is an example of one commercially available chart.

Prevention of periodontal disease

Although not all individuals with gingivitis will develop periodontitis, we currently have no means of identifying the patients that will do so. We do know, however, that individuals with clinically healthy gingivae will not develop periodontitis. Consequently, the aim is to prevent all gingivitis. This can be achieved by maintaining oral hygiene.

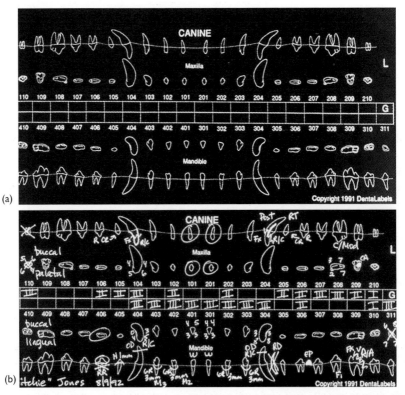

Fig. 6.1   An example of a commercially available dental chart (Canine Dentalabel): (a) blank; (b) completed.

Box 6.1 *Practical suggestions to give to owners*

- Start dental homecare as early in life as possible, as prevention of disease development is the aim. Moreover, it is far easier to train young puppies and kittens to accept dental homecare than middle-aged or older animals.
- Make the animal comfortable and approach from the side rather than in front.
- Start with just a few teeth and gradually increase the number of teeth cleaned each time until the whole mouth can be cleaned in a single session.
- The mouth does not need to be opened. It is mainly the buccal surfaces of the teeth, especially at the gingival margin, which need brushing.
- When the animal is comfortable with having the buccal surfaces of all its teeth brushed, an attempt should be made to open the mouth (by gently holding the head as far back as possible with one hand) and carefully brushing the palatal and lingual surfaces of the teeth. If this is not accepted there is every reason to continue with daily brushing of the buccal surfaces. Tongue movement helps to clean the palatal and lingual surfaces.
- Offer a reward at the end of the procedure, e.g. a game or a treat such as a rawhide strip.
- Include toothbrushing as part of the daily grooming routine. Homecare is more likely to be acceptable to an older pet if it is introduced as an extension of a pre-existing routine, e.g. evening meal, walk, grooming. Also, the owner is also more likely to remember a consistent routine.
- Owners can sit small dogs and cats on their lap whilst brushing, at the same time cuddling them to reduce their apprehension; alternatively one person cuddles and restrains whilst a second performs the toothbrushing.
- The use of a 'grooming table' type situation may be better accepted by some animals.

Maintenance of oral hygiene is performed by the owner and is, therefore, also called homecare (Box 6.1). The prevention and long-term control of periodontal disease requires adequate homecare.

The owner must also realise that, even with ideal homecare, most animals still need to have their teeth cleaned professionally at variable intervals. It is useful to draw an analogy to the situation in man, i.e. most of us do brush our teeth daily but still require dental examinations and professional periodontal therapy at regular intervals.

Maintenance of oral hygiene

The single most effective means of removing plaque is toothbrushing. Regular removal of plaque prevents gingivitis developing as well as restoring inflamed gingivae to clinical health. Studies have shown that brushing once daily will restore inflamed gingivae to health (Tromp et al, 1986b; Gorrel and Rawlings, 1996b). Clinically healthy gingivae can then be maintained by brushing three times a week if the brushing is meticulous (Tromp et al, 1986a). If brushing is less effective, then three times a week is insufficient to maintain clinically healthy gingivae. It will, however, reduce the severity of gingivitis as compared to an unbrushed control group (Gorrell and Rawlings, 1996b). Brushing once a week has not been proven to be effective in preventing or treating gingivitis (Tromp et al, 1986b).

Acceptance of toothbrushing

Most dogs and many cats will accept toothbrushing as a part of their daily regimen. It is easier to introduce the procedure to the young animal but most adult dogs will tolerate it. Cats are generally less amenable to the introduction of toothbrushing than dogs, but with patience and persistence most will accept some degree of homecare. Toothbrushing should be introduced in a gentle fashion and gradually over a period of time. Allow 3–4 weeks for the animal to accept cleaning of all teeth in one session.

Toothbrushes and toothpastes

There are innumerable brush-head and handle design and sizes available; but there is insufficient evidence to clearly commend any particular one. The choice of brush should be based on the effectiveness of plaque control in the hands of each individual. In general, a small soft to medium texture nylon filament brush seems to be the most comfortable. A flannel cloth folded over a finger, or a 'finger brush' may be more comfortable for animals and owners, but is less effective than a brush. The use of a finger brush or cloth during the training phase is useful, but every attempt should be made to get the animal to accept a proper toothbrush. The use of a non-foaming tasty pet toothpaste is recommended to facilitate plaque removal and increase animal co-operation due to its pleasant taste. The paste should be pressed down into the bristles to maintain it on the brush or the animal will just lick it off.

Brushing technique

There is no one correct method of brushing but rather the appropriate one that in each case removes plaque effectively without damaging either tooth or gingiva. A particular method must be dictated by individual preference and dexterity and the variable dentogingival morphology occurring with different stages of disease. In most instances, a combination of roll and miniscrub technique, as described in the following, will achieve the objective.

The teeth and gingival margin are brushed in a circular motion. The brush is angled at a 45° angle so that the bristles enter the gingival sulcus and shallow periodontal pockets (Fig. 6.2). Toothbrushing only cleans around 1 mm below the gingival margin. The circling motion should ensure that all cracks and crevices in and around the teeth are cleaned.

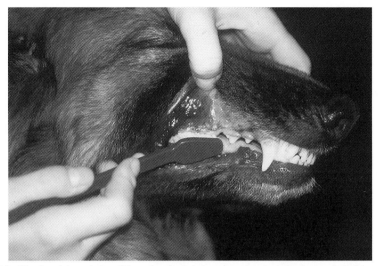

Fig. 6.2 The brush is angled at 45° so that the bristles enter the gingival sulcus and shallow periodontal pockets. Toothbrushing only cleans around 1 mm below the gingival margin.

Frequency of toothbrushing

While we know that meticulous plaque removal reduces the required frequency to every other day, most owners will not be able to achieve the standard of plaque removal required. Consequently, at our present level of knowledge, the recommendation should be daily toothbrushing.

Success of toothbrushing

For homecare to be successful the following criteria must be met:
- a motivated owner;
- a co-operative animal;
- an owner with the technical ability to perform toothbrushing.

Moreover, the effect of homecare measures must be continuously assessed and the owner's motivation continuously reinforced.

Diet and periodontal disease

The texture and form of the diet has an effect on plaque accumulation and consequently on disease development. Several studies have investigated the local effect of diet on plaque formation and development of gingivitis in the dog (Egelberg, 1965; Gorrell and Rawlings, 1996a; Harvey et al, 1996b; Logan, 1996;

Gorrell and Bierer, 1997). A coarse diet may reduce plaque accumulation on some teeth and on some tooth surfaces (Egelberg, 1965). A recent study performed over a six month period, investigating oral cleansing by dietary means, showed that dogs consuming a test diet (Prescription Diet® Canine t/d® – (Hill's Pet Nutrition Inc, Topeka, USA) had significantly less plaque, calculus and gingival inflammation than the control group (Logan, 1996). Similarly, the daily use of a specifically designed dental hygiene chew (Pedigree Rask®/Dentabone™ – (marketed in Europe as Pedigree Rask® and in the USA as Pedigree Dentabone™) reduces plaque accumulation and reduces gingivitis (Gorrell and Rawlings, 1996a; Gorrell and Bierer, 1997). There is as yet no magic bullet that we can feed our pets to prevent periodontal disease. Daily toothbrushing remains the single most effective method of maintaining clinically healthy gingivae. However, reduction of plaque by dietary means is a useful adjunctive measure and should be recommended to pet-owners.

Other adjunctive measures

The use of products aimed at encouraging chewing activity may be beneficial, by maximising the self-cleansing effect of function and physiological stimulation of salivary flow and composition. None of the products in this category is as effective as toothbrushing.

A variety of hard biscuits, rawhide shapes or strips (and other natural products, e.g. dried pig's ears, cow's hooves), rubber and nylon toys are on the market. It is recommended that dogs should be encouraged to chew these products daily, preferably shortly after eating their main meal.

The chewing of bones cannot be recommended; the hazards outweigh any possible benefits. Chewing on hard bone is likely to lead to tooth fractures, often with pulp exposure, and gingival lacerations. Softer bones are chewed and swallowed, often causing digestive problems, or become impacted on or between teeth. Raw bones are also potential sources of infection for animals and owners (*Sarcocystis, Toxoplasma, Campylobacter, Salmonella*, etc.).

Chemical plaque retardants

There are several chemical agents available on the market which claim an anti-plaque and consequently an anti-gingivitis effect. Chlorhexidine has been shown to be the most effective anti-plaque agent to date. Its main disadvantage is that it stains the teeth. Moreover, its effectiveness is reduced by the presence of organic material. So, for best results, chlorhexidine should be used in combination with toothbrushing which physically removes plaque and reduces tooth staining.

Putting homecare into practice

Before treatment is instituted, the owner must be made aware that homecare is the most essential component in both preventing and treating periodontal disease.

Whenever possible it is useful to institute a homecare programme before any professional periodontal therapy is performed.

Client education and the institution of effective homecare will, in most cases, prevent the development of periodontal disease. In the busy veterinary practice this is usually best delegated to the nursing staff, under the supervision of the veterinarian.

Client education and training in homecare techniques

Client education consists of explaining the aetiology and pathogenesis of periodontal disease. Photographs of the various stages of the disease are very effective aids (Fig. 6.3). This is followed by a demonstration of toothbrushing technique by the nurse. The demonstration should be performed on a model or skull and also on the pet. Following this initial consultation, it is essential to book a follow-up consultation a few weeks later to check the adequacy of the toothbrushing technique. The use of plaque disclosing solution can be very helpful (Fig. 6.4).

Critical timing

The ideal time for client education and training in oral hygiene measures is at the appointment for primary vaccination. The animal is given a full clinical examination and first vaccination by the veterinarian and is then passed on to the nurse. The follow-up consultation with the nurse occurs at the time of second vaccination. Following this initial training, oral health and hygiene should be checked at regular intervals. For most animals this is naturally at the time of booster vaccination. More frequent check-ups with either the veterinarian or the nurse may be necessary in certain individuals.

Marketing dental care to clients

Clients need to know about the availability of an Oral Healthcare programme and how it will benefit their pets and themselves. Marketing methods include:
- talking about it at every opportunity,
- demonstrating how the owner can examine their pet's mouth and showing clients the difference between healthy and diseased mouths,
- reception and consulting room posters,
- client information leaflets,
- articles in newsletters,
- focused mailings.

In addition, make sure appropriate toothbrushes and toothpaste arte available on sale in the reception area.

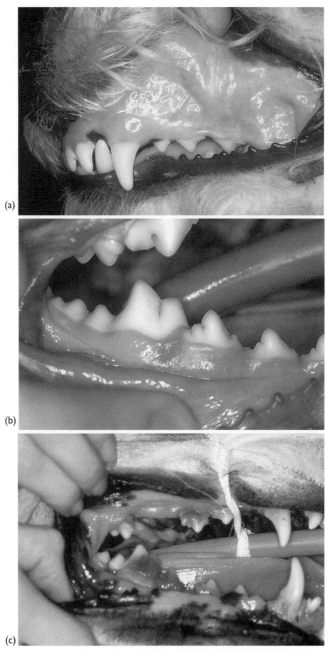

Fig. 6.3   (a) Clinically healthy gingivae; (b) gingivitis; (c) periodontitis.

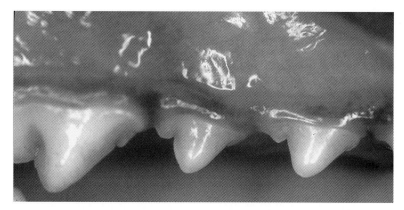

Fig. 6.4 Disclosed plaque 48 hours after professional periodontal therapy.

Treatment of periodontal disease

Professional periodontal therapy is performed under general anaesthesia and includes:
- supra- and subgingival scaling;
- root planing;
- tooth crown polishing;
- subgingival lavage;
- extraction;
- and, sometimes, periodontal surgery.

In an animal with established periodontal disease, it is vital that the professional periodontal therapy is followed up by daily homecare. However meticulous the professional therapy, if no homecare is instituted then plaque will rapidly reform. Again, employing the nursing staff to educate, demonstrate and check efficacy of toothbrushing is recommended.

It should be remembered that scaling/polishing inevitably causes a transient bacteraemia. In man, antibiotic cover for patients with valvular disease, e.g. rheumatic fever, is essential. The use of intravenous ampicillin at the time of general anaesthetic induction may be a useful precaution in animals with known valvular disease.

Feline oral diseases

Stomatitis (oral inflammation of any cause) is common in the cat. Periodontal disease is the most common cause of oral inflammation (Reichart et al, 1984; Harvey, 1995). In addition to the type of periodontal diseases seen in the dog and in man, the cat suffers from intense, chronic inflammatory reactions which affect the gingivae and mucous membranes of the oral cavity. This syndrome is known as feline chronic gingivitis–stomatitis. In a study which involved 700 domestic pet cats in the United States, inflammation which extended beyond the mucogingival line was reported in 1.5% of cats presented for periodontal or related therapy, and faucitis in 0.5% (Harvey and Shofer, 1992). In a report from an Animal Hospital in the United States which placed emphasis on preventive dental care from an early age, chronic stomatitis was found to be infrequent (Mills, 1992).

Chronic gingivitis–stomatitis in the adult cat

Clinical features

The gingivae and mucous membranes are intensely inflamed. The inflammatory reaction extends beyond the mucogingival junction and into the alveolar mucosa (bucco-stomatitis). It may also extend into the glossopalatine folds (faucitis) as in Fig. 6.5. In a retrospective study some cats presented with bucco-stomatitis without faucitis and others with faucitis without bucco-stomatitis, but all cats suffered from concurrent periodontal disease (Hennet, 1997). Consequently, gingivitis–stomatitis may well be associated with an abnormal reaction to plaque. Further work is required to investigate.

Affected animals are often intensely uncomfortable and the syndrome is frustrating to treat as conservative periodontal therapy, even in combination with oral hygiene measures and antibiotic therapy, often yields only a short-term clinical improvement.

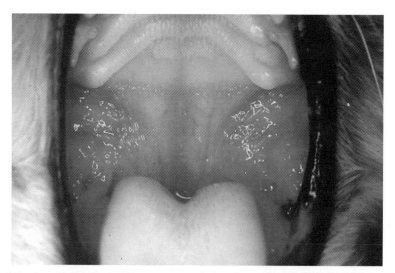

Fig. 6.5   Cat with chronic gingivitis–stomatitis with the inflammation extending into the glossopalatine folds, i.e. faucitis.

Aetiology and pathogenesis

The cause and mechanisms for disease development of this clinical syndrome remain unclear. The location of ulcerative lesions at the contact points between tooth crown and alveolar mucosa, as well as a high serum Ig against Gram-negative anaerobes, suggests that dental plaque may be a direct or indirect cause (Sims et al, 1990; Reubel et al, 1992). No specific bacterial aetiology has been identified.

Chronic gingivitis–stomatitis is characterised histologically by a cellular infiltrate where plasma cells and lymphocytes are the predominant cell types. It has, therefore, also been called plasma cell gingivitis or lymphocytic–plasmacytic stomatitis. The most consistent laboratory finding is a polyclonal hypergammaglobulinaemia. These findings suggest an immunological basis for the condition.

No specific viral aetiology has been recognized, although immunosuppressed FIV positive cats, as well as cats affected by both FIV and calicivirus, are more likely to have severe oral inflammatory disease (Knowles et al, 1989; Tenorio et al, 1990; Knowles et al, 1991; Waters et al, 1993). It has been shown that cats presenting with chronic gingivitis–stomatitis are more likely to be chronic carriers of calicivirus compared to healthy cats, and that serotypes of calicivirus isolated from cats with oral inflammatory lesions can induce acute faucitis in healthy cats (Reubel et al, 1992). However, the significance of calicivirus in the development of these lesions is still unknown.

Diagnosis

Chronic feline gingivitis–stomatitis is not a specific disease with defined diagnostic criteria. 'Diagnosis' is thus somewhat a misnomer as the diagnostic work-up is more of an attempt to confirm or eliminate possible underlying causes for the obvious intense inflammatory reactions than to reach a specific diagnosis.

Thorough physical examination and history taking permit recognition of systemic abnormalities and dermatopathological conditions. Clinical laboratory examinations are indicated, if only to exclude or confirm renal or hepatic abnormality. The total white blood cell count is very varied; a normal or increased count is the most common finding. As already mentioned, hypergamma-globulinaemia is common. Testing for FIV and FeLV is strongly recommended as a positive diagnosis may preclude further investigation and treatment in many cases.

Bacterial culture testing and antibiotic sensitivity testing is a waste of time and money. No causative bacteria or group of bacteria have been identified.

Biopsy is not rewarding in typical cases; however, asymmetrical lesions should always be biopsied as squamous cell carcinoma, the most common of oral neoplasms in the cat, may mimic the clinical appearance of a gingivitis–stomatitis lesion. Feline odontoclastic resorptive lesions (see below) may well be present concurrently and require treatment. Consequently, intraoral radiographs should be part of the diagnostic work-up.

Treatment

The initial step is meticulous periodontal therapy (supragingival and subgingival scaling, crown polishing and root planing) followed by rigorous homecare to maintain oral hygiene. Concurrent odontoclastic resorptive lesions also need to be treated (see below). Antibiotics are a useful adjunct.

Various medical treatment regimens have been advocated – for details please refer to the *BSAVA Manual of Small Animal Dentistry*, 2nd edition, 1995. However, to date, no medical treatment has been shown to give reliable long-term effects. In non-responsive cases, radical tooth extraction, i.e. removal of all premolars and molars, has led to a clinical cure in 80% of cats (Hennet, 1997).

Feline odontoclastic resorptive lesions

Feline odontoclastic resorptive lesions (variously described as feline 'neck' lesions, root resorptions, cervical line lesions, feline caries) are a common problem. The lesions should not be confused with dental caries. While early caries is a passive inorganic demineralisation of the enamel, odontoclastic resorptive lesions occur as an active progressive destruction of the dental tissues by cementoclasts and odontoclasts. The lesions occur on any tooth and anywhere on the root surface. Prevalence rates of 28.5% to 67% have been reported in the last 15 years (Harvey, 1995).

Clinical signs

Feline odontoclastic resorptive lesions are painful, and non-specific signs such as anorexia, ptyalism, jaw chattering, grinding of teeth, depression, lethargy and dysphagia may be an indication of their presence.

Aetiology and pathogenesis

The aetiology and pathogenesis of feline odontoclastic resorptive lesions is not understood.

It has been shown that periods of active resorption are followed by periods of repair of cementum and replacement of resorbed tooth substance by bone (Okuda and Harvey 1992a,b; Gengler et al, 1995; Lukman, 1996). The result is continued loss of root substance in combination with ankylosis and hypercementosis. Similar lesions have recently been reported in the dog (Bergstrom, 1992; Arnbjerg, 1996).

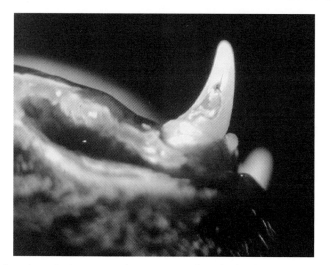

Fig. 6.6   Feline odontoclastic resorptive lesion exposing the pulp chamber.

Diagnosis

The lesions can be detected by:
- visual inspection;
- tactile examination with a dental explorer;
- radiography.

Visual inspection

The lesions most readily detected on visual inspection are those in the classical 'neck' position where they appear as cavities on the buccal or lingual aspect of the tooth. Many of these lesions are initially masked by the presence of hyperplastic gingiva or calculus deposits overlying the defect (Fig. 6.6). Detection is then only possible during a general anaesthetic after scaling the tooth surface. It has yet to be determined whether the hyperplastic gingiva is involved in the aetiology and pathogenesis of the lesion, or if it is the result of the plaque induced inflammation. The currently favoured theory is that the resorption is the initial lesion (Harvey, 1996). The defect predisposes to plaque accumulation and consequent intensification of the inflammatory response in the gingiva, resulting in the formation of the hyperplastic tissue.

Odontoclastic resorptive lesions below the gingival margin are missed on visual inspection. Moreover, it is impossible to determine accurately the extent and depth of the lesion based on visual inspection alone.

Tactile examination with a dental explorer

Tactile examination with a dental explorer may allow detection of lesions within the sulcus and a more thorough estimation of depth, but is still only a rough guide.

Radiography

More definitive diagnosis of the presence and full extent of the lesion requires radiography. Good quality radiographs viewed under magnification are necessary to detect small or early lesions. The lesions appear as radiolucent areas during periods of active resorption. During the bony replacement phase, ankylosis may start to become apparent. Often a combination of radiolucent and radiodense areas is seen.

Treatment

The aim of any treatment is to relieve pain, prevent progression of disease, and restore function. Suggested methods of managing odontoclastic resorptive lesions include:
- conservative management;
- extraction;
- coronal amputation;
- restoration.

Conservative management

Conservative management is only indicated for shallow lesions not extending into the dentine. The long-term success rate of early conservative management has yet to be determined. The follow-up must include radiographic examination.

Treatment, under general anaesthesia, consists of removing hyperplastic gingiva, followed by meticulous professional periodontal therapy (supragingival and subgingival scaling, crown polishing and root planing). The surface of the lesion is then further polished smooth to reduce plaque retention and facilitate home hygiene measures.

In instances where insufficient attached gingiva remains to make gingivoplasty possible, an apically positioned periodontal flap may be considered to make the lesion supragingival and thus accessible for homecare measures.

Topical fluoride preparations may well provide a palliative effect by hardening and desensitising cementum and dentine. It has yet to be proven that fluoride application will prevent or retard the progression of these lesions. Although topical fluoride is theoretically of benefit there is the complication that our pets will swallow the fluoride-containing agents and thus have a variable and relatively uncontrolled systemic intake with potentially harmful acute and chronic side-effects (Gorrell, 1994). As in children who swallow their toothpaste, the use of fluoride-containing toothpaste in cats is not recommended.

Good oral hygiene is recommended for the control of periodontal disease. Since periodontal disease and feline odontoclastic resorptive lesions may be linked, plaque control may slow down development and/or progression of the resorptive lesions. No studies have been reported, however, to confirm this assumption.

Conservative management as described above needs regular follow-up by means of both clinical and radiographic examination.

Extraction

Resorptive lesions which expose dentine, especially if they extend into the pulp chamber, warrant extraction of the affected tooth. In general, subalveolar resorptive lesions also necessitate tooth extraction.

Extraction of teeth with resorptive lesions can be difficult. The general principles of tooth extraction apply. Raising a mucoperiosteal flap, removing buccal bone, sectioning multirooted teeth and careful elevation of segments will allow successful extraction in the majority of cases. It is generally thought to be essential that the whole root is extracted, although this is now being questioned. Routine postoperative radiographs are necessary to assess the completeness of extraction.

Atomisation. The routine use of power equipment to 'atomise' the root is often recommended as an extraction technique for feline teeth. Atomisation may easily result in iatrogenic injuries including submucosal emphysema, other soft tissue injury, trauma to adjacent tooth roots and thermal bone necrosis resulting in sequestrum formation. This procedure should be seen as a last resort when less traumatic means of tooth extraction have failed and it is essential to remove the root remnants, e.g. inflamed pulp and ongoing periapical pathology already present at the time of extraction.

Coronal amputation

Loss of the crown and gingival overgrowth over root fragments occurs as a consequence of undetected and untreated lesions. The resulting root remnants are only detected on routine radiography and are not necessarily associated with clinical problems. Based on the above, it is suggested that complete extraction may not always be necessary. It is possible that remaining root remnants will undergo complete resorption. Alternatively, the root remnants stay embedded in the bone causing no clinical problems. This is part of the rationale behind the recent suggestion to treat this problem by means of coronal amputation (DuPont, 1995). This procedure involves raising an envelope flap to expose the cemento-enamel junction. The crown is amputated at this level and the gingiva is closed over the root remnants. It is essential that the root remnants are monitored clinically and radiographically at regular intervals. The results of this technique over a period of one year were excellent.

Some complications which can occur include periapical lesions and associated pathology in the surrounding bone, sometimes with the formation of fistulous tracts. As a rough guide, root remnants of teeth that are not endodontically compromised at the time of extraction are theoretically less likely to cause complications than those that are. Endodontically compromised roots should be completely extracted.

Restoration

Restoration has been recommended for the treatment of accessible lesions which extend into the dentine and do not involve pulp tissue. Endodontic treatment prior to restoration is necessary if the lesion is causing pulpitis or actually extends into the pulp tissue. Several studies have shown that the lesions continue to progress (Lyon, 1992; Roes and Fahrenkrug, 1993; Zetner and Steurer, 1995; Harvey et al, 1996a). Consequently, the use of restoration of feline odontoclastic lesions as a major treatment technique cannot be recommended.

Cat incisor teeth are so small that it is impractical to attempt restoration, and extraction is really the only sensible treatment.

Restoration of the premolars and molars is neither advisable nor in the best interest of the cat due to the associated technical difficulties and the progressive nature of the condition irrespective of treatment. Extraction remains the best option.

The canines are the largest and probably functionally most important teeth of the feline dentition. They are therefore the teeth where restoration may occasionally be indicated.

In summary

The purpose of the treatment is the relief of pain. The aetiology and pathogenesis of the lesions is incompletely understood, and evidence to date shows that they are progressive. Early treatment has not been proven to help long-term success. The owner must be aware of the progressive nature of these lesions and understand that the purpose of treatment is palliative and not curative and that regular clinical and radiographic examinations are required to monitor the progression of lesions that are managed conservatively. Effective homecare measures to control plaque and maintain periodontal health are required. In most instances, extraction of the tooth remains the preferable option once the lesion has exposed the dentine. Successful extraction and uncomplicated healing needs clinical and radiographic monitoring.

The importance of clinical and radiographic follow-up is even more critical in the instances where root remnants have been left in situ.

Other dental problems

The dog and cat suffer from very similar dental conditions to those seen in ourselves. These include dental caries, traumatic tooth injuries requiring endodontic and restorative therapy, and malocclusions, to mention a few. It is outside the scope of this chapter to cover these conditions. However, the benefit of homecare and frequent dental check-ups by the veterinarian is that both periodontal disease and caries can largely be prevented. In addition, with homecare these problems are identified much earlier than would otherwise be the case. This allows for earlier treatment which will reduce the degree of discomfort and pain suffered by the affected animal. The aim of veterinary dentistry is a comfortable animal with a functional bite. Aesthetic considerations are of secondary importance.

References

American Academy of Periodontology (1996). World workshop in periodontics. *Annals of Periodontology*, **1**(1), November.

Arnbjerg, J. (1996). Idiopathic dental root replacement resorption in old dogs. *Journal of Veterinary Dentistry* **13**(3), 97–99.

Bergstrom, A. (1992). Root resorption in a dog. *British Veterinary Dental Association Journal* **2**, 5.

Catanzaro, T.E. (1998) *Medical Records: Continuity of Care for Pride and Profit. Building the Successful Veterinary Practice: Programs & Procedures* (Chap. 3, Vol 2). Iowa State University Press, Ames, Iowa.

DeBowes, L.J., Mosier, D., Logan, E., Harvey, C.E., Lowry, S. and Richardson, D.C. (1996). Association of periodontal disease and histologic lesions in multiple organs from 45 dogs. *Journal of Veterinary Dentistry* **13**(2), 57–60.

DuPont, G. (1995). Crown amputation with intentional root retention for advanced feline resorptive lesions – a clinical study. *Journal of Veterinary Dentistry* **12**(1), 9–13.

Egelberg, J. (1965). Local effects of diet on plaque formation and gingivitis development in dogs. I. Effect of hard and soft diets. *Odontologisk Revy* **16**, 31–41.

Gengler, W., Dubielzig, R. and Ramer, J. (1995). Physical examination and radiographic analysis to detect dental and mandibular bone resorption in cats: a study of 81 cases from necropsy. *Journal of Veterinary Dentistry* **12**(3), 97–100.

Gorrell, C. (1994). The effects of fluoride and its possible uses in veterinary dentistry. Proceedings, 3rd World Veterinary Dental Congress, Philadelphia, USA.

Gorrell, C. and Bierer, T.L. (1997). Longer term benefits of a dental hygiene chew. Proceedings, 5th World Veterinary Dental Congress, Birmingham, UK.

Gorrell, C. and Rawlings, J.M. (1996a). The role of a 'dental hygiene chew' in maintaining periodontal health in dogs. *Journal of Veterinary Dentistry* **13**(1), 31–34.

Gorrell, C. and Rawlings, J.M. (1996b). The role of tooth-brushing and diet in the maintenance of periodontal health in dogs. *Journal of Veterinary Dentistry* **13**(3), 139–143.

Gorrell, C. and Robinson, J. (1995). Periodontal therapy and extraction technique. In: Crossley, D.A. and Penman, S. (eds) *Manual of Small Animal Dentistry*. British Small Animal Veterinary Association, Kingley House, Church Lane Shurdington, Cheltenham, Gloucestershire, GL51 5TQ, p 139–149.

Harvey, C.E. (1995). Feline oral pathology, diagnosis and management. In: Crossley, D.A. and Penman, S. (eds) *Manual of Small Animal Dentistry*. British Small Animal Veterinary Association, p 129–138.

Harvey, C.E. (1996). Are dental resorptive lesions in cats caused by dental plaque-induced gingival inflammation? Proceedings, 10th Annual Veterinary Dental Forum, Houston, Texas.

Harvey, C.E. and Shofer, F.S. (1992). Epidemiology of periodontal disease in dogs and cats. Proceedings, Annual Meeting, American Veterinary Dental College.

Harvey, C.E., Anderson, J.A. and Miller, B. (1996a). Longitudinal study on periodontal health in cats. Proceedings, Annual European Veterinary Dental Society meeting, Bordeaux.

Harvey, C.E. Shofer, F.S. and Laster, L. (1996b). Correlation of diet, other chewing activities and periodontal disease in North American client-owned dogs. *Journal of Veterinary Dentistry* **13**(3), 101–105.

Hennet, Ph. (1997). Results of periodontal and extraction treatment in cats with gingivo-stomatitis. Proceedings of the Veterinary Dental Forum **8**,49. 1994. *Journal of Veterinary Dentistry* **14**(1), 15–21.

Knowles, J.O. Gaskell, R.M., Gaskell, C.J., Harvey, C.E. and Lutz, H. (1989). Prevalence of feline calicivirus, feline leukaemia virus and antibodies to FIV in cats with chronic stomatitis. *Veterinary Record* **124**, 336–338.

Knowles, J.O. McArdle, F. and Dawson, S. (1991). Studies on the role of feline calicivirus in chronic stomatitis in cats. *Veterinary Microbiology* **27**, 205–219.

Lang, N.P., Karring, T. and Lindhe, J. (1997). Proceedings, 2nd European Workshop on Periodontology. Quintessence, Berlin.

Lindhe, J. (ed). (1993). *Textbook of Clinical Periodontology* (2nd edn). Munksgaard, Copenhagen.

Lindhe, J., Hamp, S-E. and Loe, H. (1975). Plaque induced periodontal disease in beagle dogs. A 4-year clinical, roentgenographical and histometrical study. *Journal of Periodontal Research* **10**, 243–255.

Loe, H. and Brown, L.J. (eds) (1993). Classification and epidemiology of periodontal diseases. *Periodontology 2000* **2**, 1–158.

Logan E. (1996). Oral cleansing by dietary means: results of a six-month study. Proceedings of a Conference on Companion Animal Oral Health, University of Kansas, USA, March 1–3, 1996.

Lukman K. (1996). Prevalence patterns and histological survey of feline dental resorptive lesions. Proceedings Annual British Veterinary Dental Association Meeting, Birmingham, UK, 1996.

Lyon K. (1992). Subgingival odontoclastic resorptive lesions. Classification, treatment and results in 58 cases. *Veterinary Clinics of North America* **22**(6), 1417.

Mills A. (1992). Oral dental disease in cats: a practitioner's perspective. *Veterinary Clinics of North America* **22**(6), 1297.

Okuda, A. and Harvey, C.E. (1992a). Etiopathogenesis of feline dental resorptive lesions. *Veterinary Clinics of North America* **22**(6), 1385.

Okuda, A. and Harvey, C.E. (1992b). Immunohistochemical distributions of interleukins as possible stimulators of odontoclastic resorption activity in feline dental resorptive lesions. Proceedings Annual AVDC–AVDS–AVD Meeting, 1992.

Reichart, P.A., Durr, U.M., Triadan, H. and Vickendey, G. (1984). Periodontal disease in the domestic cat: A histopathologic study. *Journal of Periodontal Research* **19**, 67–75.

Reubel, G.H., Hoffmann, D.E. and Pedersen, N.C. (1992). Acute and chronic faucitis of domestic cats. *Veterinary Clinics of North America* **22**(6), 1347.

Revert, S., Wilkstrom, M., Mugrabi, M. and Claffey, N. (1996). Histological and microbiological aspects of ligature-induced periodontitis in Beagle dogs. *Journal of Clinical Periodontology* **4**, 310–319.

Roes, F. and Fahrenkrug, P. (1993). Long-term results of glass ionomer fillings in neck lesions. Proceedings, Annual European Veterinary Dental Society meeting, 1993.

Sims, T.J., Moncla, B.J. and Page, R.C. (1990). Serum antibody response to antigens of oral gram-negative bacteria by cats with plasma-cell gingivitis-pharyngitis. *Journal of Dental Research* **69**(3), 877–882.

Slots, J. and Taubman, M.A. (1992). *Contemporary Oral Microbiology and Immunology*. Mosby Year Book, St Louis.

Tenorio, A.P., Franti, C.E., Madewell, B.R. and Pedersen, N.C. (1990). The relationship of chronic oral infections of cats to persistent oral carriage of feline calici, immunodeficiency, or leukemia viruses. Proceedings, AVDC–AVD Annual Meeting, 1990.

Tromp, J.A., Jansen, J. and Pilot, T. (1986a). Gingival health and frequency of tooth-brushing in the beagle dog model. Clinical findings. *Journal of Clinical Periodontology* **13**, 164–168.

Tromp, J.A., van Rijn, L.J. and Jansen, J. (1986b). Experimental gingivitis and frequency of tooth-brushing in the beagle dog model. Clinical findings. *Journal of Clinical Periodontology* **13**, 190–194.

Waters, L., Hopper, C.D., Gruffydd-Jones, T.J. and Harbour, D.A. (1993). Chronic gingivitis in a colony of cats infected with feline immunodeficiency virus and feline calicivirus. *Veterinary Record* **3**, 340–342.

Zetner, K. and Steurer, I. (1995). Long-term results of restoration of feline resorptive lesions with micro-glass composite. *Journal of Veterinary Dentistry* **12**(1), 15–17.

Vaccination and Parasite Control

7

Caroline Jevring

Vaccination and parasite control are two of the most important factors that have contributed to improved health and longevity of companion animals. For most practices, providing vaccinations and selling parasiticides has become the 'bread and butter' of practice income: it is so routine that these services run the risk of seeming unimportant in maintaining health. But vaccination and parasite control are vital components of modern wellness programmes. In this chapter, the contribution of vaccination to animal health is highlighted and reinforced. A brief overview of the importance of internal and external parasite control is presented, but management is discussed in detail in Chapters 3 and 11.

The importance of vaccination

If vaccinations are being used for economic rather than for health reasons, the profession would do well to condemn and remove the offenders.
Dr S. R. Nusbaum

In the United States, practices are losing their vaccine business to mail-order drug companies, human pharmacies, and pet megastores where company veterinarians adminster cut-price vaccinations. The same thing may happen, eventually, in Europe. For many practices loss of vaccine sales directly represents lost income, but if this is what veterinarians are grumbling about they have missed the point. Vaccinating a pet is a great deal more than just selling a vaccine. Vaccines should only be administered to healthy animals, so the vaccination appointment provides the ideal opportunity to talk and teach about healthcare (see later).

An erratically vaccinated population of cats and dogs is wide open to a disease epidemic. For example, inadequate vaccination schedules and/or vaccine failure are believed to have contributed to the increasing incidence of distemper and post-vaccination encephalitis in the UK since the 1960s when vaccination first radically reduced the threat of this debilitating and often fatal disease.

Why have these other sources of vaccinations been able to creep into the picture? As with most areas of preventive care, veterinarians have not done a terribly good job either of informing the pet-owning public about the importance of vaccination, or of explaining their own role in preventing disease and advising on healthcare. As a result, many owners still believe that the vaccinations given at the puppy/kitten stage give life immunity, or that geriatric pets do not need vaccinating. Some never vaccinate their pets at all. Many owners see a vaccination as an expensive procedure which requires minimal skill and so can be done by anyone.

This is supported by data: a National Opinion Poll survey in 1992 found that over a third of dogs and cats in the UK had not been seen by a veterinary surgeon in the last year. Although 78% of cat owners and 89% of dog owners said that their pets received their primary vaccinations, only around 30% of cat owners and 45% of dog owners had their pets booster vaccinated.

It is vital for the sake of animal health and owner security that veterinarians maintain control of vaccination. They must do this by getting owners to see the veterinarian as teacher and prime source of healthcare information instead of

Age	Puppy schedule for wellness	Kitten schedule for wellness
6 weeks	Physical examination *Vaccinations*: distemper/hepatitis, parainfluenza/leptospirosis, parvovirus/coronavirus *Faecal test* for parasites/deworming *Rec.* premium growth diet *Rec.* prophylactic dental care	Physical examination *Vaccinations*: rhinotracheitis, calici, panleukopenia *Testing* for feline leukaemia and parasites/deworming *Rec.* premium growth diet
9 weeks	Physical examination *Vaccinations*: distemper/hepatitis, parainfluenza/leptospirosis, parvovirus/coronavirus *Faecal test* for parasites/deworming; begin heartworm prevention *Rec.* premium growth diet *Rec.* prophylactic dental care	Physical examination *Vaccinations*: rhinotracheitis, calici, panleukopenia, feline leukaemia *Deworming* *Rec.* premium growth diet *Discuss* dental care
12 weeks	Physical examination *Vaccinations*: distemper/hepatitis, parainfluenza/leptospirosis, parvovirus/coronavirus, *Bordatella* *Faecal test* for parasites/deworming *Rec.* premium growth diet *Rec.* prophylactic dental care	Physical examination *Vaccinations*: rhinotracheitis, calici, panleukopenia, feline leukaemia, feline infectious peritonitis *Deworming* *Rec.* premium growth diet *Discuss* dental care
16 weeks	Physical examination *Vaccinations*: distemper/hepatitis, parainfluenza/leptospirosis, parvovirus/coronavirus, *Bordatella*, rabies plus a tag *faecal test* for parasites/deworming *Rec.* premium growth diet *Appointment* for spay/neuter *Rec.* prophylactic dental care	Physical examination *Vaccinations*: feline infectious peritonitis, rabies plus a tag *deworming* *Rec.* premium growth diet *Discuss* dental care *Appointment* for spay or neuter

Table 7.1   Example of how vaccination fits into wellness programmes in the United States

doctor/disease fixer, and by helping owners understand the link between regular vaccination, wellness healthcare and responsible ownership.

Gaining owner cooperation and understanding

To make it easy for owners, vaccination should be a regular part of a health schedule. How often vaccination is performed varies from country to country, even from area to area, depending on local epidemiology and disease incidence. This difference is highlighted in the examples below from America and Sweden: the incidence of all infectious diseases of cats and dogs in Sweden is generally low, and rabies vaccination is only required for pets coming into the country (this includes animals that live in Sweden who travel abroad and return to Sweden) (see Tables 7.1 and 7.2).

Owners must also understand what 'vaccination' means. A vaccination is far more than simply giving an injection in the back of the neck with a bit of

Age	Puppy schedule for wellness	Kitten schedule for wellness
Adult yearly needs	Physical examination *Vaccinations:* distemper/hepatitis, parainfluenza/leptospirosis, parvovirus/coronavirus, *Bordatella*, rabies plus tag *faecal test* for parasites (every 6 months)/deworming, routine occult heartworm test Six-month supply of heartworm preventive, Six-month supply of flea preventive *Rec.* premium life-stage diet *Rec.* prophylactic dental care	Physical examination *Vaccinations:* rhinotracheitis, calici, panleukopenia, feline leukaemia, feline infectious peritonitis, rabies plus tag *deworming* *Rec.* premium life-stage diet *Discuss* dental care Six-month supply of flea preventive
Senior health needs annually	Physical examination *Urinalysis* (specific gravity, protein) *Blood* biochemistry and haematology *Vaccinations:* distemper/hepatitis, parainfluenza/leptospirosis, parvovirus/coronavirus, *Bordatella*, rabies *Faecal test* for parasites (every 6 months)/deworming, routine occult heartworm test Six-month supply of heartworm preventive Six-month supply of flea preventive *Rec.* premium senior diet Prophylactic dental care	Physical examination *Urinalysis* (specific gravity, protein) *Blood* biochemistry and haematology *Vaccinations:* rhinotracheitis, calici, panleukopenia, feline leukaemia, feline infectious peritonitis, rabies plus tag *deworming* *Rec.* premium life-stage diet *Discuss* dental care

Table 7.1 Continued

Age	Puppy vaccination	Kitten vaccination
7 weeks	Parvovirus (*before* puppy leaves breeder)	(7–8 weeks) Rhinotracheitis/calici, panleukopenia
12 weeks	Distemper, hepatitis, parvovirus, (*Bordatella*)	Rhinotracheitis/calici, panleukopenia
First birthday, thereafter annually	Parvovirus *annually*, distemper and hepatitis *every other year*	Rhinotracheitis/calici, panleukopenia (*Chlamydia* is recommended in breeding establishments and for show cats)

Table 7.2 Recommended vaccination protocol in Sweden

colourless fluid and taking a fistful of money for it. The actual *service* the veterinarian sells is *protection* from contagious, potentially fatal diseases. Protection is nebulous – it is difficult to define, varies from animal to animal, and depends to some extent on the owner's expectations (is it total 100% protection against all diseases? is it immediate? how critical is it if they are a few days late for re-vaccination? and so on). Giving a vaccination to provide this magical 'protection' is an act of trust: the pet-owner must believe that the millilitre of colourless fluid will, in fact, provide the protection the veterinarian says it will. Implicit in this trust is that the veterinarian selects the correct vaccine, that it is the most efficacious, that it is properly stored and administered, and that it is accompanied by the correct advice.

An extremely important additional aspect of this trust relationship is that the vaccine is administered to a healthy animal. It is therefore essential for a veterinarian to perform a clinical examination of the animal, even if the owner says the animal is in full health. Immunosuppression by some drugs or by concurrent illness can reduce the immune response to the vaccine – the promised protection is not provided. The clinical examination is also an ideal opportunity to discuss other health issues with owners, and it is not uncommon to find problems that they have not noticed themselves, such as growths and dental calculus which need treating.

Interestingly, in a survey performed some years ago, clients whose pets had received a vaccination during a routine consultation were asked afterwards if they were sure their pet had been vaccinated. A surprisingly high percentage were unsure, and some were even convinced the vaccine had not been given. The lesson to learn from this is that it is very important to talk the owner through a physical examination and make it quite clear what you are doing when you give the vaccine.

Building the family–pet–vet bond

Pets age faster than humans: seeing an animal once a year can be said to be equivalent to a human going to the doctor/dentist/optometrist/chiropractor and psychologist once every 8 years. A recent American study showed that owners thought 15–20 minutes to be an ideal length of time for them to spend in the consulting room (in some UK practices, clients are still pushed through at a rate of one every five minutes!) But 20 minutes perhaps only once a year for a healthy animals is not much on which to build a sound and flourishing client relationship. Repeated annually for, say, seven years (the average life-span of an American dog), this only represents 2½ hours in a lifetime – not nearly enough time to establish the family–pet–vet bond, let alone discuss effective pet ecosystem management and healthcare issues.

A vaccination service provides an invaluable excuse to get owners in through the door: it is important that the practice then gives the client more reasons to keep coming in. Use a vaccination appointment as a base to build on: show clients how you can meet their needs for parasite control, nutritional and behavioural counselling, and dental management. Through meeting these needs you augment the family–pet–vet bond, improve pet healthcare, and increase practice income.

Communicating with owners

Vaccine companies generally produce excellent and informative booklets for pet-owners about the types and importance of vaccination for their cat or dog. It is worth highlighting the need for vaccination – both for the safety of their own animals and for the health of others with whom they have contact – every time a client brings their pet to the clinic. This can be as simple as the receptionist reading the medical journal and saying, 'Oh good, I see Flossie is up to date with her vaccinations,' to having a policy of no animals being admitted into the practice for investigative surgical or medical procedures if they are not vaccinated. All animals that are boarded, at a veterinary premises or privately, should have up to date vaccinations.

The annual booster reminder is an effective and simple way of helping clients recall when their pet should be re-vaccinated (Table 7.3). Studies show that around 60% of clients respond to the first reminder they receive, a further 20% to the second, and the remaining few can often be encouraged into the practice by a personal telephone call. An effective and well-monitored vaccination system can thus have an almost 100% recall rate, and a practice can be proud that their healthcare message is so well accepted by their clients.

Vaccination schedules for breeding establishments and boarding kennels

Where animals are grouped together, the risk of infection is increased. Veterinarians working with breeders and boarding kennels should be able to make

- As pets receive their first vaccination, fill in a booster reminder card and file it according to the month the next vaccination is due.

- Post out the reminder and check the response against a list of all who were mailed.

- Send a further reminder to those who did not respond first time. Check them off on the list when they come in for their appointment.

- Phone those clients who have still not responded asking for general information – is the address is correct, has the pet been vaccinated elsewhere (and if so, why?) and so on. This stage is best performed by someone not directly connected with the practice, and can provide a valuable source of client feedback. Remember, dissatisfied clients often don't complain – they often just don't come back! By finding out what the problem is, it may be possible to redress it in the practice.

Table 7.3 Setting up an effective vaccine reminder system

recommendations for effective vaccination schedules. For example, all animals entering a kennel or cattery should be up to date with their vaccinations; for dogs, protection against kennel cough is usually advised.

Feline leukaemia virus (FeLV) is an example of a disease of cats which has a complicated aetiology but which can be controlled by careful husbandry, isolation practices, and vaccination. Transmitted by close contact between cats, the incidence of infection varies depending on husbandry conditions and ranges from 0% in closed FeLV-negative catteries to up to 30% in FeLV infected multi-cat households. Affected cats can remain symptom-free for months or years following infection. Expression of the disease is often stress-related, and treatment is, at best, symptomatic. Control of FeLV in closed feline populations is achieved by 'test and removal' procedures. In infected multi-cat households and free-roaming cats, some protection from infection may be provided by vaccination of non-infected cats.

Summary

Annual vaccination provides immunity against and reduces spread of contagious, often fatal, diseases of cats and dogs. It provides at least a once-yearly opportunity to meet pet-owners and discuss their animal's health with them. This meeting can form the basis for a productive and profitable long-term relationship with pet-owners.

The importance of parasite control

Parasites of cats and dogs can be divided into two groups: internal ('worms') and external. Untreated heavy infestations are at best debilitating, at worst fatal. A number of parasites pose a zoonotic risk. Management of the common parasites is outlined in the chapters on *Care of the young animal*, and *The influence of environmental factors on health*.

In the United States, heartworm is a severe problem in many areas and is controlled by routine screening and prophylactic administration of oral drugs.

The key to parasite management is meticulous owner education. For example, many pet-owners still choose to buy their wormers or flea-control products from the supermarket rather than the veterinarian, on the basis that it is easier and cheaper. Unfortunately, many of these products are not very efficacious and enable infestations to build up. Taking time to teach owners about the importance of *regular* parasite management with *effective* drugs, and helping them follow sometimes taxing treatment protocols, improves pet health and reduces the risk of zoonotic infection.

References and further reading

Becker, M. (1996). 20 minutes a year just isn't enough. *Veterinary Economics* **November**, 64–66.

Catanzaro, T.E. (1998) *Building the Successful Veterinary Practice: Programs & Procedures* (Vol 2). Iowa State University Press, Ames, Iowa.

Ettinger, S.J. and Feldman, E.C. (eds) (1995). *Textbook of Veterinary Internal Medicine* (4th edn). W.B. Saunders, London.

Nusbaum, S.R. (1997). Maybe the biologic system is just flawed. *DVM Newsmagazine* **July**, 28.

Breeding and Birth Control

8

Caroline Jevring

Every year millions of unwanted cats and dogs are euthanased by veterinarians and humane societies. Systems – or lack of them – for registering pet ownership, and the sheer size of the pet population are contributory factors in this appalling waste of life but the statistical implication is that the message veterinarians have been transmitting for years about controlled breeding and birth control is not getting through to the pet-owning public.

This chapter looks at the reasons for and against neutering of pets, and also considers the role of the veterinarian in helping the novice breeder take a responsible and caring attitude towards breeding.

Neutering

Neutering is the general term for the surgical removal of the sexual organs. Ovariohysterectomy (spaying) of the bitch or queen involves the surgical removal of the ovaries, uterus and associated structures of the reproductive tract. Castration of the male cat or dog entails the surgical excision of the testicles. The operation is final and cannot be reversed.

Sterilisation by severing the male spermatic cords or female Fallopian tubes is not routinely performed in pets as it does not affect their sexual behaviour – which is often one of the primary purposes of neutering.

Owners sometimes ask about ovariectomy or hysterectomy as birth control options for their pets. These are generally not an option in cats and dogs. Ovariectomy reduces sex hormone related behaviour such as expressing heat, calling, etc., but does not eliminate the risk of pyometra. Hysterectomy does not eliminate sexual behaviour, and may induce hysteria in some animals.

Neutering can also be performed medically using oral or injectable hormone preparations such as megoestrol acetate. 'P-pills' (pregnancy prevention) or injections can be used in female animals to prevent or suppress the heat period. In males, they may be used to suppress undesirable sex-related behaviour such as territory-marking and aggression. As their effect is generally only temporary they are particularly of value in situations such as temporary heat suppression of, say, a working bitch with male companions, or to see if surgical castration would significantly affect male behaviour.

Their use has been associated with a number of negative side-effects such as reduced fertility in breeding animals, and increased incidence of pyometra. Females may become pregnant if the preparation is not given regularly or correctly, and deformed fetuses have occurred where cats continue to be dosed during an unsuspected pregnancy.

Mismating or misalliance in the dog can be controlled by large doses of injectable oestrogen. However, this is not a suitable method of routine birth control as it prolongs the heat period and there is a fairly high risk of endometrial hyperplasia and pyometra developing. There are no safe misalliance preparations for cats.

When to neuter?

The age at which these procedures should and can be performed is still debatable. Spays performed on a limited number of prepubertal bitches at a few months of age appear to have no adverse effect on bone growth or general health. Prepubertal spaying of kittens and puppies is endorsed both in the United States and the UK by many prestigious organisations including the Humane Society of America, the American Veterinary Medical Association, the American Kennel Club, the BSAVA, and BVA. They argue that operating at this age is easier, less traumatic to the animal, guarantees there are no unwanted litters, and should cost less. These are particularly important considerations for the welfare organisations who may be rehoming puppies and kittens at this age, and want to guarantee no further breeding and unwanted litters.

In practice, many veterinarians still prefer to wait until the animal is nearer sexual maturity or, in the case of females, has had its first heat. But it is not always easy to detect the first heat in either a dog or a cat, so there is a risk of them producing an unwanted litter.

Why neuter?

Neutering of pets is performed for three reasons:
1. to prevent unwanted pregnancies;
2. to prevent the development of sex-hormone related diseases of the reproductive tract and associated organs;
3. to manage or eliminate sex-hormone related behaviour.

Contraception (see above)

It has been estimated that an entire female cat can be responsible for the production of 20 000 offspring over five years. Early neutering prevents even the risk of pregnancy, the distress and expense involved in the humane disposal of unwanted kittens and puppies, and is an important aspect of animal welfare.

Medical reasons

Spaying performed before the first or second oestrus cycle in the bitch significantly reduces the incidence of mammary tumours. This effect is less marked in cats. Removal of the uterus also prevents the development of pyometra. Naturally, good surgical practice is necessary when handling viscera, in selection of suture and ligature materials, in exposure of the ovaries, and in the placement of clamps and ligatures. In one study, incomplete removal of ovarian tissues accounted for nearly half of the complications seen after surgery: others included damage to a kidney or ureter, and infection of the uterine stump.

Surgical removal of the testicles prevents the development of testicular tumours and age-associated benign prostatic hyperplasia. Testicular tumours represent up to 15% of all tumours seen in male dogs, but are extremely rare in cats. Cryptorchid dogs and dogs with inguinal testicles form a higher risk group: tumours occur 13 times more frequently and at a younger age in dogs with undescended testicles.

Behavioural reasons

Both cats and dogs show sex-associated behaviour which is more or less disturbing to their owners, neighbours, and others. This behaviour can be largely controlled or prevented by early neutering. Late neutering generally has less effect on behaviour as much of the behaviour is then learnt rather than directly hormonally related.

Male dogs under the influence of testosterone may, for example, exhibit the following behaviour:

- *Wandering.* They may wander for miles seeking bitches in heat. They create a nuisance both for the owner of the bitch and the owner of the dog itself, and are a risk for traffic accidents.
- *Aggression* towards other dogs, especially in the presence of a bitch in heat.
- *Frustrated sexuality* expressed as inappropriate mounting of people, other animals (such as the household cat), or inanimate objects.
- *'Love-sick' behaviour* expressed as howling, anorexia, restlessness and weight loss.

Tomcats tend to:
- travel long distances searching for queens in heat;
- show territorial and sexual aggression towards other (male) cats; owners of tomcats become frequent visitors at their local veterinary surgery as a result of infected fight wounds;
- caterwaul – a weird and disturbing sound which annoys everyone in the neighbourhood;
- territory mark – their urine has a pungent smell; excessive marking, especially in the house, can be very unpleasant and the smell difficult to remove.

Female animals are also affected by oestrogen and progesterone swings. Bitches may:

- show marked swings of temperament and become snappy and short-tempered around the oestrous period;
- leave bloody marks all round the house during their heat;
- show broody or 'nesting' behaviour associated with false pregnancy;
- lactate, sometimes heavily, with the associated risk of developing mastitis,

Queens may:

- call piercingly and almost continuously during their heat;
- show extra affection by rubbing against people or objects and/or writhe on the floor so that owners sometimes think they are having a fit;
- develop a false pregnancy with or without milk production;
- disappear in search of males.

Behaviour is multifactorial: it can be changed by manipulating the environment, altering the physiological status of the animal via surgical techniques and drug therapy, or using learning principles such as behaviour modification techniques. Neutering is one method of altering undesirable sex-hormone related behaviour, but it is not necessarily the best or only option in managing all problem cases, especially in older animals.

Responsible pet ownership and pet behaviour

People often have illusory and unreal expectations of companion animals, knowing and caring little about their basic needs and natural behavioural tendencies. Human reaction to reversion to instinctual behaviour – so-called 'inappropriate behaviour' – ranges from distaste to terror. The interest of dogs in eating and rolling in all sorts of insanitary matter disgusts many owners. Reports of domesticated town dogs gathering in packs to attack and even kill children are shocking and disturbing.

Pets are unable to live their natural lives within the constraints of human society. As in caring for children, an adult with responsibility for a pet cannot surrender that responsibility in a permissive ideal of natural *laissez-faire*, i.e. the misguided 'naturalism' of letting dogs be dogs, allowing them to run free, breed indiscriminately, and so on. A pet must be protected. A relationship without responsible ownership is contrary to the contemporary socioecological ramifications of pet ownership. While some owners may need to be educated towards greater empathy with their pet, others need to be taught about greater responsibility.

Emotional factors underlie many cases of apparent irresponsible ownership (see Table 8.1), as opposed to indifference or ignorance. For example, an owner may identify his or her own sexuality in the companion animal and therefore see neutering of it as a personal threat. Men generally don't like the idea of castration, for example, and women question the need for a total ovariohysterectomy.

Owner's reasoning	Source of idea	Support for reasoning
She needs a litter of puppies/kittens to be fulfilled	Outdated concept from human psychology that women need to have babies to be 'fulfilled'	None. There is no evidence female animals *need* to have young
She/he should be allowed to lead a natural life	See above: can reflect owner's own attitude to sexual freedom	None: rather, reflects owner's lack of responsibility and/or understanding of pet's natural behaviour
She/he will become fat	Neutered animals tend to gain weight more easily	True: can usually be easily controlled by attention to diet and exercise, especially in obese-prone breeds
It'll affect his/her personality	Because neutering is used in some cases to manage behaviour problems, many owners assume pets will become 'neutral' and lose their personality	Personality is based on far more than the effect of sex hormones. Neutering may calm an excited animal, reduce aggression and other sex-related behaviour but it does not influence the true personality of the pet
He'll be less of a dog – and he'll know it	Some (male) owners are concerned that male dogs will lose their 'maleness'. Some also claim their dogs are 'sad' as a result of castration	These and attitudes reflect human worries about themselves. Implantation of 'neuticles' (prosthetic testicles) usually resolves owner (and dog) worries
It's great for the kids to see where babies come from	Children should experience life's processes at first hand	A debatable point: yes, it's a great experience for most children, but on the other hand it represents more pets to find caring, responsible owners for, plus an often surprisingly heavy investment of time and money
It'll affect her coat		Some bitches experience coat changes after spaying, especially spaniels
The breeder says we ought to breed from him/her	Owners of quality pedigree animals sometimes enter contracts with the breeder where by they promise a number of puppies/kittens back to the breeder	The veterinarian should discuss the advisability of breeding from pedigree animals just because they are pedigree

Table 8.1 Common owner reasons for not neutering their pet

Owner's reasoning	Source of idea	Support for reasoning
We can make some money on a litter		Implies a total lack of responsibility. In addition, not all pregnancies are problem free, litters may be small, and the costs of rearing may be much greater than expected. New owners also have to be found
It costs too much to spay	Owners look simply at the cost not the benefits	Cost-saving benefits of spaying include: it's a one-off operation, it is final – there is no risk of subsequent pregnancies, there are no expenses involved with pregnancies and unwanted offspring, it reduces the risk for mammary tumours (see above) and eliminates the risk of pyometra
Tradition	'I've never seen the need, and I've kept dogs for years'	In some countries, such as Sweden, there is not the tradition of neutering. Most pets are well controlled and, until recently, it was illegal to spay a bitch on non-medical grounds. However, the shockingly high level of pyometra that followed this law means that it has now been withdrawn

Table 8.1   *Continued*

The owner of a young bitch in heat recently phoned me in tears. 'What shall I do?' she begged. 'She's out in our garden now, tied to a tree being mated. I've been so careful all through her heat. I don't want her to have puppies.'

I explained to her about misalliance injections and, in fact, she subsequently agreed to spaying. In the meantime, I phoned the owners of the male dog in question – he was the father of several litters in the area – and gently suggested that perhaps they should either keep him confined or consider castrating him. 'We're not castrating him,' his male owner replied. 'He has a right to live as he wants.'

'But what about the bitch he's just raped – in her own garden.'

'That's her owner's problem. She shouldn't allow her dog out when she's in heat. It's irresponsible!'

Emotional factors cannot be used as the basis of an argument for letting a pet live a 'natural' life as it impinges on the rights of others in society. A lonely dog that barks continuously, or a tomcat that sings on the neighbour's fence, is a nuisance. The options for the owner include pet-training, surgical or medical intervention, rehoming, and euthanasia. Of these, early neutering is often the simplest and most effective option.

Unfortunately, it is not only pet-owners and breeders who argue against neutering of pets. It is also veterinarians. Knowing the medical risks associated with, in particular, not spaying females, I think this borders on negligence.

Talking to owners

Talking to owners about neutering as the most effective method of birth control can start even before they get their pet. It should certainly be discussed when the owner first presents the new pet for examination; written information about what neutering involves and why it is done can be provided in the New Owner (Puppy/Kitten) pack.

The staff team should be quite clear about the contraceptive options available for cats and dogs, and be able to discuss their risks and benefits knowledgeably with owners.

Advising about breeding

Some owners elect to breed from their pedigree pet through a planned mating. Advice about breeding and care of the bitch/queen is an issue veterinarians often leave to breeders – partly because veterinarians are expected to focus on contraception as part of responsible pet ownership, and partly because they often lack experience themselves. Although the serious breeder is probably the best qualified person to recommend suitable matches between two pedigree animals to enhance desirable characteristics based on an intimate knowledge of their show and performance achievements, veterinarians are missing out if they are unable to advise the novice breeder about correct nutrition during pregnancy and lactation, vaccination, parasite control, what to expect during the birth, aftercare of the mother and offspring, and so on.

The first issue the veterinarian needs to be able to discuss with the owner is *why* they want to breed from their animal. When arguments like those outlined in Table 8.1 arise it may be better to recommend neutering, but if there is apparently more serious interest in having a litter, veterinarians should be able to present a balanced view of the challenges of breeding quality animals against finding homes for a large litter. Many people, for example, do not realise the costs involved in time and money in raising a litter and finding homes for them all. Convincing an animal owner that their animal is not worth breeding from can also offer a challenge in tact as most owners cannot see their animal as anything other than perfect, even if this may be a long way from the truth.

> *Presented with a young Golden Retriever bitch that the owners didn't want to spay because they wanted a litter of puppies from her, I had the difficult task of trying to point out to them that even to my relatively non-expert eye she was a very poor example of the breed. She was small, so broad across the forehead her eyes were almost on the side of her head, and had an overshot mouth. I wasn't even sure if these 'faults' could be remedied by careful selection of a suitable male.*
>
> *'But she has a wonderful temperament,' was their reply. Unfortunately I never saw them again.*

Veterinarians have a responsibility to advise owners about breeding healthy animals (see Chapter 10) but it can be difficult to maintain a professional neutrality when there is a strong feeling that a more extreme breed should probably not be bred from at all! However, if veterinarians frighten clients away, they are forced to turn to less well informed sources and the result may be very inferior quality animals.

Ideally, veterinarians and breeders should co-operate and share experience and knowledge to ensure that the animals receive the best care, and the owners accurate advice. Sadly, co-operation has often been difficult because of a resistance to recognise and acknowledge professional competence on both sides. Goodwill and the desire to listen and learn from each other can give very positive rewards (see Chapter 10).

Giving advice on general care

Basic reproductive data are given in Table 8.2.

As part of their 'womb to tomb' involvement in pet wellness there is much general advice about pre-conception care through to weaning that veterinary practices can provide. Planning an organised programme of pre- and post-partum care is the most effective way of disseminating information and working with the owner. The care can be spread over a number of surgery visits leading up to vaccination of the new litter. Some practices may prefer to recommend home visits to young litters because of the risk of infection.

Both male and female pets should be given a thorough physical examination before breeding to ensure they are well and of normal weight. Animals that are significantly over– or underweight may experience reduced fertility. Breeding problems can be referred to colleagues who have specialised in companion animal reproduction.

Vaccinations should be up to date, and the animals should be checked and treated for internal and external parasites. This is especially important for the breeding bitch/queen as a larval stage of the *Toxacara* species they harbour is activated by pregnancy. *T. cati* primarily infects kittens by intramammary transmission, *T. canis* infects puppies transplacentally. Shortly before the animal gives

Parameter	Dog	Cat
Type of reproductive cycle	Two heat periods per year	Seasonally polyoestrous
Onset of puberty	6–10 months in small breeds 18–24 months in large breeds	Mixed breed cats 5–8 months Pedigree cats 4–18 months Later in males than females Influenced by season of birth
Duration of oestrous cycle	Average 18 days	About 3 weeks Variable in pedigree cats
Oestrus	Average 9 days (range 3–21)	Around 7 days
Ovulation	Generally 2 days after onset of oestrus but can be very variable	Induced ovulator Ovulation about 36 hours after mating
Gestation	64 days (range 56–72)	63 days (range 59–70)
Litter size	Average 4–6 (range very wide especially in large breed dogs)	Average 4 (range 2–8)
Weaning	28–30 days	35–42 days

Table 8.2 Basic reproductive data for the dog and cat

birth it should be introduced to a suitable maternity box placed in a warm, quiet, draft-free area of the house. The box will be used for both birthing and nursing.

Nutritional requirements during pregnancy and lactation

Reproduction draws on body reserves of nutrients. With a large litter, the nutritional demands of pregnancy and lactation can be enormous. Malnourishment of the bitch/queen before and during gestation may be an important contributory factor in mortality of offspring. Clinical signs associated with feeding low quality food to bitches/queens through gestation and lactation are:

- appearance of poor condition – the animal is underweight with poor coat quality;
- uncontrollable diarrhoea during lactation because the mother is forced to eat large quantities of poorly digestible food to try and meet her energy requirements;
- 'fading puppy/kitten' syndrome;

- lactation problems;
- anaemia in both mother and offspring.

The majority of maternal weight gain occurs in the third trimester of pregnancy in the dog. In cats, there is a linear increase in body weight throughout the pregnancy. This is apparently caused by early deposition of fat tissues as post-partum body weight does not return immediately to pregestational weight as it does in bitches.

A premium quality growth/lactation type commercial diet can be fed to bitches and queens throughout the pregnancy but is most important during the last three to four weeks and throughout the lactation. Meals may need to be divided into several smaller portions over the course of the day for a bitch, especially if she is carrying a large litter. Cats tend to snack-feed anyway, eating up to 16 little meals a day when fed free-choice. Foetal size increases rapidly in the last trimester; this should be reflected in a gain in weight by the bitch/queen of around 20–25% by the time of the birth.

Often a bitch refuses food during the 12 hours prior to parturition.

Lactation presents one of the most severe tests of a diet's nutritional adequacy. The mother must eat, digest, absorb and use very large amounts of nutrients to produce sufficient milk to support the rapid growth and development of several offspring. A lactating bitch fed free-choice should be able to maintain her body weight.

If at optimal weight at whelping, a bitch/queen with an average to large litter generally requires the following amounts of food during lactation:

- first week: 1.5 times the amount needed for maintenance;
- second week: 2 times maintenance;
- third week to weaning: 3 times maintenance.

The mother of a very large litter may need more.

Fresh water should be available at all times.

Before and during weaning, restricting the amount of food consumed by the bitch can help reduce the discomfort that may arise from excessively swollen mammary glands. Once the puppies are weaned the bitch should be fed enough for her maintenance.

If a premium quality growth/lactation type diet is fed, supplementation with nutrients such as fats, minerals and vitamins is strongly contraindicated.

Feeding of the weaned puppy/kitten

Puppies are generally weaned at 3–4 weeks of age, kittens at 6–8 weeks. They often start to eat solid food before they are weaned by having access to the mother's food. If the mother is fed a premium quality growth/lactation type diet this is ideal to wean the youngsters onto. There may be an advantage to soaking kibbles to soften them in the beginning, but within a week or so the puppies/kittens should be able to eat dry kibble. Once the diet has been selected, feed only that diet. Supplementation with meat, table-scraps, or other items creates faddy eaters. Supplementation with protein, minerals, and vitamins is strongly contraindicated.

Feeding of an appropriate growth diet can continue until the puppy/kitten reaches around 90% of its adult weight, when it can be converted onto a quality maintenance type food.

House-training and hygiene

In the first few weeks of life, the mother takes care of her offspring's hygiene. Thereafter, puppies can be kept on material such as newspaper which is frequently changed, and kittens need access to a litter box. It can be quite fascinating to watch a queen seriously teaching her kittens how to use a litter tray and how to groom themselves.

Conclusion

Surgical neutering is the contraceptive method of choice for dogs and cats. It also reduces sex-hormone related behaviour and reduces the risk of some diseases occurring.

When owners elect to breed from their pets veterinarians can co-operate with breeders to provide a comprehensive wellness care programme for the parents and offspring.

References and further reading

Concannon, P.W. (1995). Reproductive endocrinology, contraception and pregnancy termination in dogs. In: Ettinger, S.J. and Feldman, E.C. (eds) *Textbook of Veterinary Internal Medicine* (4th edn). W.B. Saunders, London.

Johnston, S.D. (1995). Breeding management of the bitch. In: Ettinger, S.J. and Feldman, E.C (eds) *Textbook of Veterinary Internal Medicine* (4th edn). W.B. Saunders. London.

Preventing Canine and Feline Behaviour Problems

9

Sarah Heath

Behaviour problems are the primary reason for euthanasia of dogs between weaning and maturity in the United States. The situation is similar in the UK, and, in addition, hundreds if not thousands are rehomed or abandoned, placing an enormous strain on rescue organisations. It is the same story with cats: their increasing popularity also increases the impact of their behavioural problems, and more and more healthy cats are rehomed or euthanased.

A disease outbreak that caused such dramatic loss of life within the canine and feline populations would stimulate drug companies and the veterinary profession to work round the clock to find a cure and to produce a vaccine, but, until recently, the devastation caused by behavioural problems has met with extraordinary apathy from the veterinary profession.

The UK Association of Pet Behaviour Counsellors (APBC) noted in their annual report in 1990 that the majority of the 3000 canine cases seen by Association members over the last twelve months could have been avoided had the pet been adequately and appropriately socialised and habituated during the early weeks of life. No one is better placed than the veterinarian to offer sound and practical advice on behaviour problem prevention and decrease the number of unnecessary deaths. After all, members of the profession have an unrivalled level of access to puppies and kittens in their formative weeks via the breeder and the new owners.

Fortunately, this crucial area of preventive medicine is now one of the most rapidly expanding fields within veterinary practice as veterinarians realise that the study, recognition and treatment of behaviour problems amongst domestic pets is not only possible but is also often astonishingly simple and successful.

The need for providing a behavioural service

How many veterinarians have experienced the puppy who wriggles and bites when his toe-nails are being clipped, or the kitten that paws and scratches during auroscopic examination of the ears? The veterinary practice is an environment where behavioural problems often first come to light. Many directly affect the veterinary surgeon as he or she tries to carry out even the simplest of examinations.

Behavioural confrontation in the consulting room increases stress and the risk of injury for all concerned. It is undesirable for the practice staff and leads to an unnecessary increase in their work load because of extra time wasted on essentially simple procedures. It also increases the expense to the owner as the pet often needs sedation to be examined or medicated.

Providing a behavioural service has numerous benefits both for clients and the practice:

- improving the quality of life for animal and owner;
- increasing client appreciation of the practice;
- making life easier in the consulting room;
- increasing job satisfaction for both veterinary surgeons and nurses;
- encouraging a greater rapport with clients.

In addition, it is an area of work that can involve all members of the practice, provide a valuable extension of the veterinary nurse's role, and prove profitable. Let's look at some of these advantages in more detail.

Providing preventative behavioural medicine is an ethical necessity on welfare grounds. The veterinary surgeon's vow on admission into the Royal College of Veterinary Surgeons is that 'my best endeavour will be to ensure the welfare of animals committed to my care'. Welfare includes both the physical and mental well-being of animals.

But it is not just the welfare of the pet that is at stake – the owner's well-being is also affected. Modern small animal veterinary practice is founded on the human–animal bond. Most behaviour problems disrupt the bond and reduce the pleasure of pet-ownership. When behavioural problems push the relationship to breaking point, owners often turn to the veterinary practice in desperation. If no appropriate advice is available the animal is rehomed or euthanased. A family loses a pet, or an elderly person loses a companion – and the veterinary practice has certainly lost a client. These clients tell their friends about their bad experience.

Clients represent income: offering behavioural advice creates both direct and indirect income. Direct income comes from behavioural consultations, including supplying literature and behavioural training aids for pets who develop behavioural problems. Indirect income derives from the pleasure of owning well-behaved animals: devoted owners in a flourishing relationship with their pet are more likely to spend time and money on healthcare for their pet and they also buy pet accessories. Their dogs and cats will probably have longer life-spans compared to problem pets and generate more income for the practice over their lifetimes through regularly receiving routine healthcare. These are the good clients! They are what the practice wants!

Common behaviour problems

There has been a tendency for behavioural problems to be categorised, but this approach runs the risk of over-simplifying what are often very complex problems of multifactorial origin. The resulting 'recipe book' treatment programmes for behavioural disorders are potentially impractical and dangerous. Animals presented for behavioural consultations often display a number of behaviour problems: the selection and successful application of a treatment programme depends largely on the environment in which the individual lives and on the ability of the owner to implement the programme. Each case is therefore different. Treatment is founded on multidisciplinary principles of behaviour modification.

One of the most simple and useful ways of categorising behaviour problems for the veterinary surgeon in general practice is:
- species-typical behaviour that is considered inappropriate;
- behaviour problems that are symptoms of an underlying medical cause;
- behaviour problems for which there is no recognised medical cause.

Species-typical behaviour that is considered inappropriate

Teaching clients about the normal behaviour of their pets is a valuable component of a preventative behavioural service. Pets are often rejected because of behaviour that is perfectly normal for that species but for which the owner was unprepared. Examples of this include the need for cats to sharpen their claws, and to mark territory by urine spraying, or for dogs to dig and bury objects, or to seek out and ingest animal faeces and other unappealing matter (see *Working with prospective owners* and *Working with new owners*).

Behaviour problems that are symptoms of an underlying medical cause

No animal should be 'treated' for a behavioural condition unless it has first been seen by a veterinary surgeon. When an animal presents with behavioural changes it is essential that physical causes are excluded. This category highlights the need for strict control of non-veterinary behavioural counsellors and close cooperation with the veterinary profession.

When an animal presents with a change in behaviour a thorough medical history should be obtained and physical examination performed. When a medical condition is suspected it may be necessary to obtain further information such as results from a neurological examination, and/or blood tests (biochemistry and haematology), urine analysis, and radiography/ultrasound. More specialised tests such as ECG or CSF analysis may be performed if necessary.

Veterinary surgeons referring behavioural cases to non-veterinary colleagues must remember that the animals remain under their care. A close dialogue must be maintained between the veterinary surgeon and the behavioural counsellor to ensure that the animal receives the best possible treatment. Referral for behavioural problems should be taken as seriously as referral within any other veterinary discipline.

Behaviour problems for which there is no recognised medical cause

This category includes those behavioural problems best dealt with by preventative behavioural programmes involving breeders and prospective and new owners. Contributing factors include:

- detrimental genetic influences;
- inadequate and/or inappropriate early socialisation and habituation;
- inappropriate present environment;
- exposure to one or more traumatic experiences;
- lack of behaviour-related training;
- learning through inappropriate reinforcement.

Offering a preventative behavioural service to breeders

Veterinary surgeons should work closely with the breeders in their area, not just on medical problems and disease prevention, but also on the subject of puppy and kitten behavioural development. Many dog breeders come to their veterinary surgeon for advice about conditions such as hip dysplasia on their breeding programmes, but will not ask about maintaining good temperament in their

---

Box 9.1   Advice for breeders on socialisation and habituation

- Temperament is important in a breeding programme. Temperament of both dam and sire need to be considered, especially in feline breeding where, for example, the paternal effect on the behavioural characteristic of boldness is well documented.
- Once a litter has arrived, ensure that the puppies and kittens become accustomed to being handled in an appropriate manner. Handlers must not distress the dam.
- Gradually increase the amount of contact with people. Start with people known to the dam and gradually introduce less familiar people, as well as a wide range of individuals old and young, male and female. Take adequate precautions at all times to prevent introduction of disease.
- Encourage new owners to come and visit their pet in the breeding environment as often as possible before they take it home.
- Introduce the puppies and kittens to a wide range of environmental stimuli, including everyday household noises such as washing machines, even if it is only for a few hours a few times a week. Failing this, breeders can use tape recordings of common sounds such as children playing, doorbells, vacuum cleaners and tumble driers.
- Provide a wide range of sensory stimulation through provision of species-appropriate toys and activities, and exposure to human-related stimuli.
- Design buildings in a breeding establishment not only to take into account disease prevention and ease of management, but also appropriate behavioural development.
- Inform prospective new owners of the importance of continuing the socialisation and habituation process in the new home.

breeding lines. Similarly, they may seek veterinary advice on kennel design in relation to disease spread, but information about the effects of environment on the behavioural development of puppies is seldom sought.

The same applies with cat breeders: disease considerations usually dominate the breeder's policy decisions and the kittens' behavioural development is not considered. Offering an appropriate service to breeders takes time and a willingness from both sides to discuss matters, as well as a thorough understanding of the developmental requirements of puppies and kittens.

The sensitive periods when socialisation and habituation are believed to be crucial to successful behavioural development are between 4 and 14 weeks in the dog and 2 and 7 weeks in the cat. A significant portion of the puppy's sensitive period coincides with the period of breeder care. For many kittens, and all pedigree ones, this stage of development occurs entirely whilst it is at the breeder's premises. Veterinary practices must therefore teach breeders about the importance of socialisation and habituation (see Box 9.1).

Working with prospective owners

Pet selection service

One of the most important and, sadly, least common services that the veterinary practice can provide is advice on pet selection. Inappropriate choices often lead to early surrender of pets to rescue societies or, worse, euthanasia as the owners elect not to 'pass the problem on to someone else'. Often it is not the animal itself that is the problem, but the combination of *that* pet and *that* owner in *that* situation.

If you offer a pet selection service, advertise it clearly. Many owners are unaware that veterinary practices have *anything* to offer about pre-purchase advice. Display information about pet selection interviews to emphasise the importance of the decision-making process and encourage prospective owners to think carefully about the issues involved. This is a chance for the veterinary nurse to make a valuable contribution to the overall preventative healthcare programme in the practice by guiding prospective owners through the question process and giving them suitable advice.

An example of the sort of information that potential pet-owners should be asked to provide is given in Box 9.2. Part A deals with general background information focusing on real issues such as the amount of time and money that the owners have to spend on the new pet, and the conditions in which the pet would be expected to live. Part B considers the actual choice of pet.

Breed selection

There is a huge selection of dog and cat breeds from which to choose. Advising clients on breed selection is difficult. Although it may be possible to narrow down

---

Box 9.2   *Conducting a pet selection interview*

Part A: General questions to ask prospective owners
- Why do you want a pet?
- What particular role(s) do you want your pet to fulfil? e.g. companion, playmate, guard, rodent controller, etc.
- What specific requirements do you have for your pet? e.g. good with children, hunting companion, talking bird, competition standard.
- What is the composition of your household in terms of pets and people?
- What are the time schedules of you and your family? e.g. work commitments, school, holiday patterns.
- How much time every day could you realistically spend on your pet? e.g. for exercise, play, grooming, general care.
- What, in general terms, is the financial position of you and your family? *(This is important when considering how much you can afford to pay for the purchase, upkeep and possible veterinary costs of your pet.)*
- Where do you live? In a flat/house? In the country/town? Are you near appropriate exercise areas for a dog? Do you have a safe garden?
- Are there any special health considerations in your family? e.g. asthma, allergies, physical disability.
- What previous experiences of pet ownership do you and your family have?

Part B: Specific information about the the pet
- What type of pet do you want? e.g. cat, dog, small mammal, bird, etc.
- What breeds have you considered? (Consider adult size, colour, coat length, etc.)
- What sex of pet would you like? Why?
- What age of pet would you like? e.g. adult, kitten, puppy.
- Where had you thought of getting your pet from? e.g. breeder (professional or private), rescue centre, puppy farm, pet shop.

---

the choice according to size, coat length, exercise requirements and potential medical considerations, it is more difficult to advise specifically on behavioural parameters. Certain breeds are associated with certain behavioural traits, and some breeds are considered more suited to certain environments than others, but breed-specific generalisations are risky as behaviour development is so multifactorial. However, the veterinary profession can learn to recognise behavioural characteristics of different breeds and their suitability for different environments.

Knowledge about the origins of the breed, type (e.g. hound, terrier, utility) and the original function gives a basic indication of likely behavioural characteristics. The lugubrious nature of a St Bernard, for example, would not suit the active person seeking a sporty companion; a young male Doberman would not be a suitable companion for an elderly, infirm lady; a Jack Russell that loves digging would be a problem for a person passionate about their garden, and so on.

Behavioural characteristics of different dog breeds

A number of surveys have looked at the behavioural traits of different breeds and attempted to group together breed characteristics that appear to hold true for most individuals. For example, a survey by the Anthrozoology Institute at Southampton University grouped the 49 most common dog breeds in the UK according to certain behavioural traits. The survey asked 13 questions that covered the following traits: excitability, watchdog behaviour, snapping at children, playfulness, aggression towards other dogs, general activity, obedience training, excessive barking, dominance over the owner, destructiveness, demand for affection, ease of house-training, and territorial defence. From these questions three behavioural factors were established:

- *aggressivity* – a tendency to aggression and/or dominance;
- *reactivity* – which included demand for affection
- *immaturity* – a tendency to remain puppy-like even when the dog is adult.

The survey divided the 49 breeds into eight groups depending on their scores on the three factors; the results are shown in Table 9.1.

Information such as this is only a guideline for behaviour (Fig. 9.1). It is essential that owners remember that the way a dog behaves is determined largely by its upbringing and training. Any dog needs a great deal of early socialisation and habituation together with suitable training and care to become a sociable family

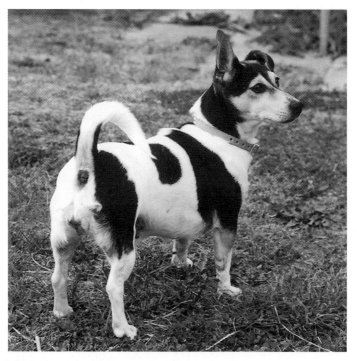

Fig. 9.1 Different breeds have different, more-or-less predictable behaviour characteristics. It is important to help prospective owners choose the breed or type of dog that will best suit their personal and family circumstances. © Ann F. Stonehouse.

Group	Characteristics	Typical breeds	Other breeds
1	Aggressivity – *high* Reactivity – *average* Immaturity – *low*	Rottweiler, German Shepherd, Doberman	Bull Terrier
2	Aggressivity – *high* Reactivity – *average* Immaturity – *high*	Jack Russell, Corgi, Cocker Spaniel	West Highland White Terrier, Cairn Terrier, Fox Terrier, Border Collie
3	Aggressivity – *average* Reactivity – *low* Immaturity – *low*	British Bulldog, Chow	Great Dane, Airedale
4	Aggressivity – *average* Reactivity – *high* Immaturity – *low*	Toy and Miniature Poodles, Yorkshire Terrier, Chihuahua	Papillon, Miniature and Standard Dachshunds, Pekingese, Lhasa Apso, Pomeranian, Shih Tzu
5	Aggressivity – *low* Reactivity – *average* Immaturity – *high*	English and Irish Setters, English Springer Spaniel	Golden Retriever, Dalmatian, Labrador, Boxer
6	Aggressivity – *low* Reactivity – *low* Immaturity – *low*	Greyhound, Basset Hound	Whippet, English Pointer
7	Aggressivity – *low* Reactivity – *high* Immaturity – *low*	King Charles Spaniel, Cavalier King Charles Spaniel	Shetland Sheepdog
8	Aggressivity – *average* Reactivity – *average* Immaturity – *average*	Samoyed, Standard Poodle, Rough Collie, Old English Sheepdog, Miniature Schnauzer, Beagle, Border Terrier, Staffordshire Bull Terrier and Scottish Terrier	None

Table 9.1   Breeds according to behavioural characteristics

pet. Any dog has the potential to develop behavioural problems, and behaviour differences between the various breeds are only a starting point. Most breeds can fit into a wide range of different life-styles provided that owners have enough knowledge, care, time and patience to succeed.

Veterinary practices are in the ideal position to offer a pet selection advice service, stocking literature on cat and dog breeds and advising prospective owners on where to find additional information (see Appendix 2).

Breed selection for cat owners

The first question that potential cat owners need to ask themselves is whether they want a purebred cat, a crossbred or a good old-fashioned moggie (Table 9.2). Making this decision can be far from easy and many owners will want to know the potential advantages and disadvantages in each case. Although choosing a cat is a very personal thing, some guidelines can be offered and the veterinary practice is in an ideal position to offer this advice in pet selection clinics.

If the owner decides to choose a pedigree kitten the choice may be overwhelming, so clients should be encouraged to ask for advice.

Very little work has been done on the behavioural traits of cat breeds, and, in comparison to dog owners, potential cat owners generally have far less information available to help them with the decision about which breed to purchase.

The behavioural profiles of four of the most common feline breeds – Siamese, Burmese, Persian, and Abyssinian – were described by Hart (1979) based on characteristics identified by a number of cat show judges associated with either the Cat Fancier's Association or the American Cat Fancier's Association. The judges emphasised that there are great differences between individuals of the same breed, and that breed generalisations may be not be true for every cat.

Cat type	Advantages	Disadvantages
Purebred	Able to predict adult characteristics in size, coat type, and even behaviour to some extent	Expensive and, depending on the breed, may have to wait for kittens to be available
Crossbred (two purebred parents but two different breeds)	Can combine desirable aspects of both breeds	May be expensive if the start of a 'new breed'. May not be readily available. Cannot reliably predict characteristics and may see the undesirable characteristics of both breeds
Moggie	Inexpensive and readily available. Wide selection of appearances, coat lengths, coat colours, etc.	Unable to predict adult characteristics and, importantly, adult behaviour. Paternal effect on behaviour is very important – in most moggies identity of the father is unknown

Table 9.2 Types of cat

The behavioural characteristics of some more unusual breeds, including the Manx, Himalayan, Russian Blue, and Rex, have also been described (Hart, 1980). Other authors have labelled further breeds with specific behavioural traits and interestingly there is broad general agreement between them, but it can be said that very little sound scientific research has been done to validate the findings. Table 9.3 attempts broadly to describe the behavioural characteristics of several cat breeds. It

Shorthairs

Siamese:
- Demanding of attention and affection
- Outgoing and confident
- Intelligent
- Become strongly attached to owners
- Highly vocal
- Good pet for children as long as they are gentle

Burmese:
- Demanding of attention and affection
- Playful extroverts
- Plenty of energy
- Easy going
- Good family pet, good with active but gentle children
- Fond of physical interaction
- Vocal but less so than Siamese

Abyssinian:
- Shy
- Fearful
- Wary of strangers
- Too nervous for children
- Intelligent and inquisitive
- Affectionate with owners but not a lap cat
- Sociable with other cats
- Quiet

Russian Blue:
- Gentle
- Affectionate
- Undemanding
- Quiet

Korat:
- Playful
- Lively
- Intelligent
- Quiet

Table 9.3 Behavioural characteristics of cat breeds

Havana:
- Demanding of attention and affection
- Intelligent
- Not very vocal

Bengal:
- Quick, agile
- Intelligent
- Very sociable
- Rarely vocalises but has a gravelly voice

Ocicat:
- Sociable with people
- Devoted to owners
- Affectionate
- Not very sociable with other cats
- Moderately quiet

Oriental shorthair:
- Energetic
- Intelligent
- Lively
- Demanding of attention and affection
- Vocal

American Shorthair:
- Unassuming cat
- Moderately loud voice

Manx:
- Sweet natured
- Undemanding
- Devoted to owners
- Playful
- Occasionally withdrawn

Longhairs

Persian:
- Lethargic
- Reserved
- Inactive
- Placid
- Undemanding
- Not a lap cat

Himalayan Persian:
- Intermediate personality between Persian and Siamese
- Lively
- Quiet and melodious voice
- Sweet natured

Table 9.3 *Continued*

Semi-longhairs

Birman:
- Intelligent
- Lively
- Charming
- Mix well with children and animals
- Loving to owners
- Sweet natured

Ragdoll:
- Laid back personality
- Moderately vocal
- Affectionate
- Playful

Somali:
- Playful
- Sensitive
- Vocal but not noisy
- Affectionate to owners

Turkish Van:
- Intelligent
- Like water
- Home-loving
- Adaptable
- Melodious voice

Balinese:
- Extrovert
- Very lively
- Extremely vocal

Rex

Cornish Rex:
- Agile
- Apprehensive
- Withdrawn
- Active
- Unpredictable
- Quiet

Devon Rex:
- Extrovert
- A monkey in cat's clothing
- Quite strident

Table 9.3 *Continued*

is compiled from several sources and can be useful as a general rather than a definitive guide for prospective owners.

Age of the pet

The decision whether to choose a young puppy or kitten or an adult animal is an individual one. Important factors include the age of the prospective owner, the time schedule of the owner, and their financial resources. The major advantage of taking on a youngster straight from the dam is that the owner can influence the pet's development right from the start and can also witness the transformation from youngster to adult. However, caring for puppies and kittens in their early life can be more time consuming than caring for an adult or even an adolescent. Choosing an older animal usually reduces concerns about house-training, but there may be a higher risk of the animal developing behavioural problems associated with the after-effects of poor training. If owners are determined to take on a mature animal they should be encouraged to obtain as much information as possible about the animal's previous homes and they should be advised to adopt only via a reputable rescue organisation.

The best age to bring a kitten or a puppy home will depend on the level of socialisation and habituation provided by the breeders. If breeders are behaviourally aware and have paid adequate attention to the behavioural development of the kittens or puppies in their care then the decision about the age for rehoming is not as crucial as when the environment in which the youngsters are being raised is devoid of suitable stimulation.

It is generally recommended that the best age for rehoming puppies is 6–8 weeks in order to ensure that they have a good level of socialisation with their own species, and have learnt from their dam and litter mates before entering a human world. It is very important for the puppy to continue to gain experience in canine communication once it leaves the litter, which is where puppy parties and playgroups come in (see later).

Kittens can be rehomed at around eight weeks of age, with the exception of pedigree kittens who are required to remain with their dam until they are fully vaccinated. The much earlier sensitive period of socialisation and habituation for kittens (from between 2 and 7 weeks of age) means that the onus for their development during this period falls on the breeder (see Chapter 3).

Sex of the pet

Owners' expectations have as much to do with the choice of sex of the pet as they have with the animal itself. Preferences for male or female cats are not as strong as for male or female dogs but most owners have preset ideas about which sex they would prefer. The value of generalisations – such as that male dogs are more likely to be aggressive, female dogs are easier to train, male cats are fighters and female cats are more home loving – is limited. Male and female cats and dogs can make equally rewarding pets.

The issue of neutering is one that owners need to consider carefully (see Chapter 8). Castration of male dogs reduces the sexually dimorphic behaviours such as roaming, urine marking, mounting and some forms of aggression, while castration in cats is strongly associated with the control of indoor urine spraying, fighting and roaming. The behavioural advantages of spaying are not so well documented in either species but, on the grounds of health and responsible pet ownership, neutering is advisable if the owner has no plans to breed from the pet. It is important to advise clients about the pitfalls of breeding and to emphasise that it is not something to be undertaken lightly. Breeding should not be considered if there is *any* medical or behavioural problem with the pet.

Source of the pet

The best sources of cats and dogs are reputable breeders, either private or professional, or well-organised and well-run rescue organisations. Obtaining a pet

---

Box 9.3   *Advice for prospective owners choosing a puppy or kitten*

- Do not underestimate the work involved in caring for a new puppy or kitten. Carefully consider your choice of pet: species, breed, age and sex are all important. Be realistic in your expectations concerning financial and time commitments.
- Do not purchase your kitten or puppy from a pet shop or from an outlet that claims to sell a range of different breeds.
- Take the time to locate a reputable breeder or visit a reputable rescue organisation. Be prepared to travel some distance if necessary.
- Ask to meet the dam and, if possible, the sire.
- Spend time observing the litter at play and watching how they interact.
- Look for a litter where all of the puppies or kittens are outgoing and confident.
- Observe the behaviour of other animals at the breeder's premises or visit owners of dogs and cats from previous litters as this will give an indication of the success of socialisation and habituation programmes carried out by the breeder.
- Observe reactions by the puppies or kittens to novel stimuli in their environment such as a new toy, and to strange and unexpected sounds such as the gentle rattling of car keys. Normally the puppies or kittens should appear surprised but quickly recover and go to investigate.
- Handle the puppies or kittens and see their reaction to strange people. The way in which a young animal responds to being handled and examined gives a good indication of the success of socialisation.
- Once you have selected a kitten or puppy arrange to visit it as often as possible prior to collection in order to build up a relationship with your new pet.
- Do not be too impressed with immaculate and clinically clean premises if they are totally devoid of stimulation. Cleanliness is important but so too is habituation.

direct from the breeder has the advantage that the owners can see the dam and often the sire and other siblings. They can also follow the puppy or kitten's progress from birth to the time of adoption.

Buying kittens or puppies from pet shops or from an outlet that sells a range of different breeds should be strongly discouraged (Box 9.3). In many cases puppies and kittens from these sources have been bred in totally unsuitable environments and are at risk from a range of medical and behavioural problems. Unfortunately, some prospective owners feel that they have a 'duty' to rescue these animals from their appalling conditions; the veterinary practice can point out that although one individual may have been rescued, buying these puppies and kittens has the unfortunate side-effect of perpetuating the process and ensuring that more animals will suffer. Clients need to understand that the only way to stop unscrupulous people from trading is for everyone to refuse to buy their pets.

Taking on an older animal from a rescue centre can be very rewarding, but there are many rescue centres whose only concern is a rapid turnover of animals. Animals enter a vicious circle of recycling where they spend their lives going from rescue centre to new home and back again. Prospective owners should be advised to use only those rescue organisations that have a good reputation for matching animals and owners, and who are able to offer appropriate advice for people accepting animals with behavioural problems and needs (Box 9.4).

The role of temperament testing

General temperament evaluation can be made by observing puppies and gauging their relative activity levels, playfulness, excitability and general health.

Box 9.4   *Advice for prospective owners choosing an adult pet*

- Where will you get your pet from? If you are considering a rescue animal, visit the rescue centre some time before you make your decision about your pet: check their facilities and ask about their rehoming policy.
- Resist the temptation to take an animal home on impulse. Do not base your selection purely on appearance – there is a lot of information that you need to know first.
- Find out as much as possible about the animal's previous history, about the environment in which it lived and the human composition of its previous household.
- Be patient in the early stages after adoption, but start as you mean to go on. *Consistently* apply the house rules that you wish to establish.
- Expect a honeymoon period – it can take three or four weeks for behavioural problems to show.
- Do not fall into the trap of selecting an adult rather than a puppy or kitten because they are 'less work' – this is not necessarily true.

Individual evaluation can be carried out by separating a puppy from the rest of the litter and observing its reactions in a range of situations, for example being groomed, having its nails trimmed, being lifted up, and having food or toys removed.

The puppy aptitude test (PAT) is often used in the selection of puppies. There is a considerable amount of controversy over its validity and value, but bearing in mind its limitations, it is a useful tool in pet selection.

The testing determines the *current* temperament of the animal in situations of fear, sociability, excitability and reaction to handling; it is not necessarily a reliable predictor of adult behaviour. Its usefulness lies primarily in identifying inappropriate behaviours and indicating the existence of *early* problems, which enables the breeder to address the situation promptly and to carefully select an owner who is both willing and able to provide the appropriate handling. *Failure* to display inappropriate behaviour during the temperament test does *not* guarantee that behaviour problems will not develop.

The PAT gives a measurable score and is usually carried out between 7 and 8 weeks of age. It is performed on one puppy at a time by a tester that the puppy has never met before, in an environment with few if any distractions. The traits assessed in PAT include social attraction to people, sound sensitivity, touch sensitivity, response to restraint, response to physical control, stability and energy level. If prospective owners are told about the PAT score for their new puppy they need to be aware of its limitations.

Evaluation of the temperaments of kittens is less well researched. The personality of the father is known significantly to affect that of the kitten, but often the identity of the father is unknown. Three common feline personality types have been identified in the cat:

- shy, timid and unfriendly;
- confident, outgoing and friendly;
- active and aggressive.

It is estimated that as many as 15% of cats may never be able to be socialised successfully enough to make good pets. In general, shy, aggressive and withdrawn feline individuals are best avoided as potential companions.

It is sensible for prospective owners visiting kittens, prior to purchase or adoption, to observe the litter at play and to watch the interactions between the queen and her offspring. Shy or aggressive behaviour or signs of boldness and friendliness may be significant. Handling the kitten is important to test its reaction to being lifted up, stroked, and brushed. Clients should be wary of situations where the breeder insists on picking the kitten up and holding it while the prospective owner has a quick stroke! Finally, prospective owners should observe how the kittens react to novelty in the form of strangers or unexpected noise. None of these tests gives any accurate prediction of the cat's behaviour later in life but they can be helpful in sounding warning bells for inappropriate behaviours.

Working with new owners (see Chapter 3)

Advising owners about the prevention of behavioural problems in dogs and cats, and offering practical help to dog owners via puppy parties and playgroups are some of the effective ways the practice can provide preventative behavioural management. The advantages are many:

- helping in the prevention and early identification of behavioural problems;
- fostering the principles of responsible pet ownership;
- encouraging early rapport with both clients and patients;
- enhancing the importance and value of the human–pet bond;
- helping new owners develop a better understanding of their pets;
- resulting in better behaved adult pets who are an asset to the community and a pleasure to have as patients on the practice books;
- increasing opportunities for the practice to inform their clients about additional services;
- a lot of fun for both the practice staff and the owners and their pets.

The vaccination programme and behaviour

At the crucial time when puppies should be socialising, maternal immunity is waning and the risk of disease increasing. Veterinary surgeons must balance the need for disease prevention through vaccination and limited contact with potential disease sources such as other animals and 'the street', with that of adequate opportunity for normal psychological development. For many years this created a social vacuum for puppies. Now it is possible to fully protect puppies and kittens from infectious diseases by early vaccination and still cater adequately for their psychological needs (see Chapters 3 and 7).

Puppy parties

Puppy parties were first advocated by veterinarian Dr Ian Dunbar in the late 1980s and are now hugely popular in veterinary practices round the world. His idea was to gather a group of new puppies, their owners, and families together for a party where they could be taught about how to care for their pet, including highlighting the importance of socialising their puppy both with other dogs and with children. Puppies find children exciting. If children do not learn what to do and what not to do at an early stage the puppy may develop aggression and biting problems. Puppy parties are thus an excellent way of building rapport with clients whilst highlighting the importance of responsible pet ownership (Box 9.5).

Puppy parties are easy to organise and are a perfect forum for veterinary nurses who can run the parties and answer the questions that new puppy owners regularly ask about behaviour and training (Box 9.6).

The small cost of providing puppy parties should be seen as an investment in good client relations – which will continue through the pet's life – and good public relations, which can only be beneficial for the practice's image within the local community (Box 9.7). Many companies are only too pleased to sponsor these events in return for the opportunity to introduce their products to receptive new puppy owners.

There are many benefits to running puppy parties (see Box 9.7).

Box 9.5 *Basic protocol for organising puppy parties in your practice*

- Held on one evening per month.
- Puppies attend between 9 and 12 weeks of age (between first and second vaccinations).
- Each puppy only attends one party.
- Up to 8 puppies at each party.
- All of the family are invited, especially children, as the presence of a wide range of age groups helps provide valuable socialisation for the puppies.

The party lasts for about one and a half hours and it is free to clients. The practice provides safe suitable toys and tiny tit-bits for the puppies, and soft drinks and light refreshments for the owners. At the end of the evening each puppy receives a party bag to take home in which there is an edible treat and a selection of leaflets giving information about the practice and the services it offers including behaviour management, dentistry and nutrition.

Box 9.6 *Basic format for a puppy party*

The actual format of the evening depends on the practice but generally the party begins with an introduction from the staff and a period of socialisation. Owners are shown how handle their own puppies correctly – including training their puppy to accept daily examinations of its feet, teeth, eyes and ears – and are then encouraged to handle all of the other puppies in a game of 'pass the puppy'.

Next, owners learn about preventive healthcare topics and how to put behaviour in a health and welfare context. Issues covered include:

- parasite control
- nutrition
- neutering
- vaccination
- prevention of behaviour problems.

Puppies are then taken individually into a consulting room and introduced to the veterinary surgeon/nurse who gives the puppy tit-bits and gentle handling while the puppy is standing on the table. This helps to form pleasant associations with the consulting room and makes consultations in the future far less traumatic for pets and their owners as well as for the veterinarian.

This is followed by a short period of play where owners are taught the importance of playing the right games. Finally, owners are given the opportunity to ask questions.

Box 9.7 *Benefits of running puppy parties*

To owners:
- Opportunity to meet with other puppy owners
- Chance to talk in detail with veterinary practice staff
- Learning about their pet's development
- Better behaved pet who is a pleasure to own

To pets:
- Opportunity for socialisation with other dogs and people
- Chance to form positive associations with the veterinary practice and its staff
- Better education and training from owner
- Decreased need for chemical restraints for simple procedures

To the practice:
- Opportunity to develop closer relationship with clients
- Opportunity to promote principles of preventive health-care
- Better behaved animals in the consulting room
- Chance to market other practice services to clients

Puppy socialisation classes

As a follow-up to a puppy party, owners are advised to enrol their puppies in puppy socialisation classes. These classes are the very earliest form of training for puppies. They are usually run as a 4–6-week course and provide the opportunity for appropriate socialisation and hands-on training. Many veterinary practices have the facilities to set up puppy classes and veterinary nurses have taken on this area of work very successfully.

Where practices need to recommend external puppy classes they should first screen the classes carefully as the way in which they are run is crucial to their success. Inappropriate socialisation and habituation experiences at this critical stage can cause the development of behaviour problems rather than their prevention. The products of unsuccessful puppy classes can end up in behavioural clinics later in life. For example, free-for-alls with large numbers of puppies being let off to 'enjoy themselves' can do more harm than good. The temperaments of the puppies present need to be taken into account: nervous, withdrawn individuals should be given the opportunity to explore without being overwhelmed by others. Periods of off-lead socialisation need to be controlled.

Establishing links with trainers

Basic obedience training is a vital key to a good dog–owner relationship and has a strong role to play in the prevention of behavioural problems. It is not usually

145

possible or appropriate for veterinary surgeries to offer training classes at their premises, but they can provide owners with information about local trainers. Again, care should be taken with recommendations.

Kitten evenings

The popularity of puppy parties has demonstrated just how receptive new owners are to information and help. Kitten owners are no different, and with the increasing popularity of the cat many practices are now finding that they have a higher percentage of cat than dog owners as clients.

Socialisation and habituation are as important for the successful behavioural development of the kitten as they are for the puppy and yet kitten owners traditionally receive a fraction of the help and support available to puppy owners.

At the first International Veterinary Behaviour Meeting in 1997, Dr Kersti Seksel described her Kitten Kindergarten programme in Australia. Briefly, she invites kitten owners to attend two one-hour 'kitten kindy' classes a week apart to learn more about feline behaviour and healthcare. These classes are not simply feline versions of the puppy party since cats and dogs are two very distinct species and the methods appropriate for socialising dogs do not apply for cats. Classes are limited to 3–6 kittens and each kitten must have had its first vaccinations. Kittens older than 14 weeks are excluded as they may simply learn to fight rather than play unless the classes are very well controlled. The aims of the classes according to Dr Seksel are fourfold:

- to increase the knowledge of owners about cats;
- to have better behaved adult cats;
- to prevent behaviour problems;
- to build a strong bond between the veterinary practice and the client.

During classes, owners are given information about normal cat behaviour and are taught how they can influence and modify the behaviour of their pet. The kittens play with suitable toys and explore and develop confidence in strange surroundings (Fig. 9.2). They are never forced to interact and cardboard boxes are provided for those kittens who would rather hide! The owners are taught the principles of training their pets through using rewards, and the appropriate use of rewards and discipline are discussed in detail. The importance of environmental enrichment for totally indoor cats is emphasised: owners are shown how to compensate for the lack of opportunity to display normal feline behaviours outdoors. In addition to the behavioural topics, issues such as neutering, vaccination, dental care and nutrition are also discussed, and owners are encouraged to ask questions.

Kitten kindergartens are still very new and debate continues over their validity and practicality, especially from a disease point of view. However, there is no reason why kitten owners cannot be invited to to the practice *without* their pets for a 'kitten information evening'. These evenings are highly successful as a public

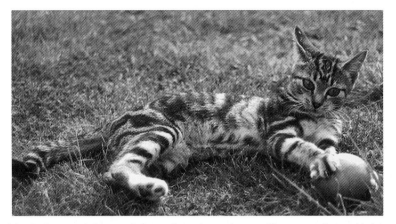

Fig. 9.2 Both cats and dogs need plenty of stimulating play time. This is part of normal behaviour. © Ann F. Stonehouse.

relations exercise and offer the opportunity for practice staff to share information about kitten development and healthcare. An adult cat or demonstration kitten can be used to show the various training techniques and handling skills, before encouraging owners to practise with their own pet at home. A kitten evening is a good compromise and shows cat owners that cats are valued by the practice as much as dogs!

The role of the owner

For any preventative behavioural advice to be successful it is essential that owners understand their own role in shaping their pet's behaviour.

Natural canine and feline behaviour

Until owners understand the basics of natural canine and feline behaviours they will be unable fully to appreciate their pet's behaviour or differentiate between what is normal behaviour in an inappropriate context and what is abnormal (Fig. 9.3). Offering information sheets about natural behaviours can be helpful. An alternative is to stock and sell behaviour books (see Recommended further reading for clients at p. 194).

Basic training using rewards

Basic training is important for both puppies and kittens. The principles of reward-based training using the lure–reward technique can be taught in a routine consultation. Teaching the puppy in front of the owner is a powerful lesson for the

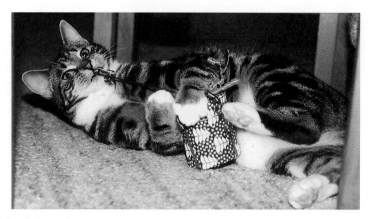

Fig. 9.3 Understanding normal behaviour gives an insight into the development of abnormal or unacceptable behaviour. Owners must be made aware of the link between the two and given help to prevent the latter developing. © Ann F. Stonehouse.

owner and an ideal chance to demonstrate the right and the wrong way to use rewards. It also gives the chance to highlight the risk of inadvertently rewarding the wrong behaviour (see Box 9.8).

You can then highlight the two very important principles involved:

- A behaviour will be learnt more quickly if the animal performs it voluntarily rather than being forced – this is more effective than the old-fashioned approach of pushing down on the puppy's bottom and forcing it to sit.
- The timing of reward is crucial if the correct behaviour is to be rewarded – if the puppy starts to get up from the sitting position as the reward is given then it is the act of getting up that is being rewarded and not the act of sitting.

This second principle is especially important: many undesirable behaviours develop as a result of such inadvertent learning. Explaining this makes owners aware of their own influence on their pet's behaviour and in the establishment of inappropriate behaviours such as jumping up, being over-exuberant in play, and barking excessively.

Box 9.8 *Demonstrating basic reward training: Sit!*

The method is simple and gives the owner a technique for taking control of their pet in a positive manner from the very beginning. Show an owner how to teach their small puppy to Sit! by raising a food reward slowly over the puppy's head until it moves naturally into Sit! position. As the puppy sits, the owner is told to say the word Sit! and *immediately* give the reward, ensuring that the puppy's bottom is *actually in contact* with the floor as the *reward is consumed.*

The role of punishment

Punishment is one of the most over-used and misunderstood methods of training. Owners need to learn how and when to use punishment, if at all. The concept of punishing wrong behaviour comes from the human misconception that the opposite of reward is punishment: the opposite of reward is *absence of reward*. Rather than punish an animal when it steps out of line, owners should be encouraged to ignore unwanted behaviours and concentrate on rewarding what is right.

Pets, like children, should be given every opportunity to succeed. They should be provided with appropriate outlets for their natural behaviours, such as digging or scratching, so that the behaviour can be channelled in an acceptable form. They should be supervised as much as possible and offered guidance at every turn. It is the owner's responsibility to engineer the situation so that the young puppy or kitten has maximum opportunity to behave appropriately and minimum opportunity to get it wrong. When it does prove necessary for the owner to intervene, for example when the young pet's behaviour is actually potentially dangerous, remote forms of punishment such as loud noises are always preferable to direct punishment from the owner.

Physical punishment runs a high risk of inducing a wide variety of behavioural problems such as hand shyness, submissive urination, fear, and even aggression. Sadly, pets are frequently seriously psychologically damaged through the inappropriate use of such physical punishment. The human hand should always be a sign of positive interaction for a pet. Owners must learn that if they hit their pet they seriously threaten their relationship.

Behaviour problems in the older animal

A lot has been written about dealing with behavioural development in young animals and preventing the development of problems at an early age, but far less information is available about the behavioural changes associated with old age. Statistics suggest that behavioural problems account for a high level of euthanasia in dogs under two years of age, and most canine behaviour problems become apparent to owners within the first few years. Cats are also more likely to be referred for behavioural problems at a young age. However, the level of tolerance of problems appears to be higher amongst cat owners and it is not unusual for cats to be older before the owner decides to eventually seek help.

Cats and dogs over the age of 10 referred to behaviour clinics present a different profile of problems. Older dogs tend to be referred with problems associated with elimination, fears, phobias and separation, whilst older cats often exhibit restlessness at night, excessive vocalisation, 'depressed' behaviour and elimination problems.

In addition to behavioural problems, owners of older animals need to be prepared for behavioural changes which are part and parcel of the ageing process. Geriatric changes within any of the major body systems can have behavioural effects. Deterioration in sight, hearing and mobility is likely to affect the behaviour of the individual, and in many cases owners notice alterations in behaviour patterns before anything else.

Changes associated with ageing are usually progressive and irreversible and owners often need counselling. Management of geriatric behavioural changes such as cognitive dysfunction in dogs depends on an accurate diagnosis of any concomitant medical problems as well as identification and, if possible, removal of any specific stimuli that contribute to the problem. Changes in the animal's environment may be needed, especially in cases involving impaired hearing or vision. Behaviour modification can be just as successful in geriatric cases as in the younger animal and the same basic principles apply even if the actual techniques must be somewhat adapted. Learning has taken place over time so patience is a very important requirement when dealing with behaviour problems in older animals. Owner education may also be needed to modify their expectations of their pet.

Behavioural counselling

In an ideal world, all of the preventative behavioural techniques would be instituted at every stage in every pet's life. The result would be a population of problem-free pets, happy owners and scar-free veterinary surgeons/nurses! Reality is different. Despite the wealth of knowledge on preventing behavioural problems, puppy farms still exist, puppies still spend the crucial weeks of their lives isolated because of out-dated vaccination programmes, kittens still fail to be socialised adequately before 7 weeks of age, and people continue to select pets that are totally unsuitable for their life-style and environment. Too many pet dogs and cats develop behavioural problems that are as life-threatening as any lethal disease.

A preventative behavioural service is an essential part of veterinary practice but it needs to be complemented by a behavioural *counselling* service for when things go wrong. It is simply not possible to provide that service within the practice in many cases, but with an ever-growing number of reputable behavioural counsellors across the UK, and around the world, the effective use of referral should mean that no animal or owner is denied the chance to tackle and resolve a pet behavioural problem.

The methods of treating behavioural problems are based on the multiple disciplines of ethology, learning theory, human psychology and veterinary psychopharmacology. The details of these methods are beyond the scope of this book but, for those veterinary surgeons who wish to expand the behavioural service that their practice provides, advice is available in other texts, some of which are listed in the references and further reading list.

References and further reading
Askew, H. (1996). *Treatment of Behaviour Problems in Dogs and Cats.* Blackwell Science, Oxford.

Beaver, B. (1992). *Feline Behaviour – A Guide for Veterinarians*. W.B. Saunders, Philadelphia.

Bradshaw, J.W.S., Goodwin, D., Lea, A.M. and Whitehead S.L. (1996). A survey of behavioural characteristics of pure-bred dogs in the United Kingdom. *Veterinary Record* **138**, 465–468.

Cargill, J. (1994). Temperament tests as puppy selection tools. *Dog World* **April**, 40–49.

Dunbar, I. *Sirius Puppy Training … the Video*. Distributed by Parkfield Entertainment, Unit 12, Brunswick Industrial Park, Brunswick Way, New Southgate, London, N11 1HX.

Hart, (1984). *The Pet Connection*. CENHARE, U of MN, Minneapolis, MN.

Hart, (1988). *The Perfect Puppy: How to Choose Your Dog by Its Behaviour*. W.H. Freeman & Co., NY.

Hart, B. L. and Hart, L. A. (1985). Selecting pet dogs on the basis of cluster analysis of breed behaviour profiles and gender. *Journal of the American Veterinary Medical Association* **186**(11), 1181–1185.

Heath, S. (1994). Providing a behavioural service in veterinary practice. Proceedings of the WSAVA Congress, Durban.

Landsberg, G., Hunthausen, W. and Ackerman, L. (1997). *Handbook of Behavioural Problems of the Dog and Cat*. Butterworth-Heinemann, Oxford.

Neville, P.F. and O'Farrell, V. (1994). *Manual of Feline Behaviour* (2nd edn). British Small Animal Veterinary Association, London.

O'Farrell, V. (1992). *Manual of Canine Behaviour*. British Small Animal Veterinary Association, London.

Overall, K. (1994). Temperament testing and training – do they prevent behavioural problems? *Canine Practice* **19**(4), 19–21.

Overall, K. (1997). *Clinical Behavioural Medicine for Small Animals*. Mosby, St Louis.

Peachey, E. *Running Puppy Classes*. Available from APBC. PO Box 46. Worcester, WR8 9YS, England.

Reisner, I. (1991). Pathophysiological basis of behaviour problems. *Veterinary Clinics of North America Small Animal Practice* **21**(2), 207–224.

Seksel, K. (1997). Kitty Kindy. *The Proceedings of the First International Conference on Veterinary Behavioural Medicine* CABTSG/ESVCE, p 28–30.

Useful addresses

Companion Animal Behaviour Therapy Study Group
c/o Mr DS Mills BVSc MRCVS
CABTSG Secretary
De Montfort University, Lincon
Caythorpe Court
Caythorpe
Grantham
Lincolnshire

European Society of Veterinary Clinical Ethology
c/o Dr J Dehasse DVM
129, Avenue de la Fauconnerie
B-1170, Brussels
Belgium

Tel/Fax: 00 32 2 675 8666
Association of Pet Behaviour Counsellors
257, Royal College Street
London
NW1 9LU
Tel/Fax: 01386 751151
E-mail: apbc@petbcent.demon.co.uk.

American Veterinary Society of Animal Behavior
c/o Dr Debra Horwitz
AVSAB Secretary/Treasurer
Veterinary Behavior Consultations
253 S. Graeser Rd
St Louis
MO 63141
USA

Animal Behavior Society
c/o Dr Ira Perelle
ABS
Mercy College
Dobbs Ferry
NY 10522
USA

Breeding for Health

10

Caroline Jevring

'Benny' is a 5-year-old male English Bulldog. He is described by his breeder as an excellent example of his breed.

Benny is very brachycephalic and breathes stertorously and laboriously even at rest. He also suffers chronic, severe dental disease related to the malformation of his jaws. The health problem for which he is most regularly treated is chronic pedal furunculosis which is controlled by his veterinarian and owner through strict hygiene, corticosteroids, and antibiotics as needed. At the age of two, his tail was amputated because of unresponsive tail-fold dermatitis. As he is unable to exercise normally, he has a tendency to be overweight.

Benny really exists, an example of the extreme physical characteristics demanded for some breeds. Dog and cat breeding has enabled people to create a great number of breeds to suit their demands for size, shape, coat, temperament, and performance. However, breeding purebred animals specifically to fulfil various purposes also makes people responsible for their health and vitality. It is not only breeders who have responsibility, it is owners, show judges and veterinarians. In this chapter the importance of these different roles is discussed, and the Swedish model for successful genetic health schemes is presented.

Origin of companion animals

Domestication of wild animals began slowly and gradually about 12 000 years ago. Dogs descended from wolves or wolf-like creatures, and dog-like remains have been found in association with human remains in a wide diversity of geographic locations from this period. From 6500 BC the dog is found virtually everywhere with prehistoric and human remains. The man–dog association probably arose from the similarity of the hunting and scavenging practices of both humans and wolves or dogs: both species are co-operative hunters working in social units that communicate with facial expressions and body postures. Selective breeding for temperament, appearance and other characteristics over many thousands of years resulted in specialised types of dog. By 2000 BC specific types of dog that perform specific jobs can be identified, from the long-legged Saluki type, to short-legged herding and hunting dogs. Within the past 100 years the diversity of breeds has increased sharply, caused in part by increased access to remote areas of the world. There are now over 400 breeds recognised by the Kennel Clubs.

Domestication of the cat is more recent than that of the dog, the wild forerunner being the African wild cat. Worshipped as a deity in Ancient Egypt, by the Middle Ages in Europe the cat had become a creature of Satan and was frequently burned, killed or buried alive as part of religious rituals to drive out the Devil. Useful for rodent control on board ship and in the colonies, cats spread to the Americas in the seventeenth century, and later became popular housepets in the nineteenth century because of their fastidious and clean habits. Now there are around 100 different breeds of cats, although the 'mog' is still the favourite.

Breed development

With dogs, breeds evolved mainly to serve a specific function which in many cases no longer exists. Papillons, for example, were developed as body warmers in the courts of the Japanese Emperors and became a convenient size to keep up the sleeves of a flowing kimono. Sharpeis were Chinese fighting dogs, their extra skin folds serving to protect them during a fight. Dalmatians were stylish carriage dogs, running beside horse-drawn carriages to protect the occupants from footpads and highwaymen. English Bulldogs were used for bull-baiting, their flat noses enabling them to grip onto an enraged bull, maintain the grip and breathe at the same time. Breeds like this are now at risk of becoming the victims of selection for extreme physical characteristics and/or focus on appearance because they are no longer 'limited' by their functional needs.

Papillons and toy breeds in general tend to suffer dystocia and dental disease related to their large domed skulls and disproportionately tiny jaws. Sharpeis are known as the 'dermatologist's dream'. Dalmatians suffer deafness related to the piebald gene for coat colour. Bulldogs can barely walk, let alone breathe. Compare these with breeds like the Greyhound, Rottweiler, Springer Spaniel or Australian Cattle Dog. These dogs are still bred primarily for an active purpose – racing, controlled aggression, tracking and mouthing abilities, and herding instinct respectively. They have to be physically and mentally sound to fulfil these roles. Problems arise with this category when they are kept as pets and the traits for which they have been bred for many generations are suppressed. Greyhounds tend to chase and kill any small creature that runs. Rottweilers may attack innocent bystanders whom they see as a threat to 'their' family or home. Spaniels' hunting instincts may mean they cannot be let off the lead during a family walk in case they disappear on some trail. Cattle dogs that herd by nipping the heels of errant cattle can inflict nasty bites on people or other animals when they try to 'herd' them.

With cats, the wide variety of breeds reflects selection for beauty rather than function. Extreme beauty is not without its problems. Persian cats, for example, suffer constant tear overflow and staining related to their desirably concave faces; Siamese cats suffer strange neuroses. Fortunately, the popularity of the 'mog' tends to mean that fewer breed-related problems are seen in cats (Fig. 10.1).

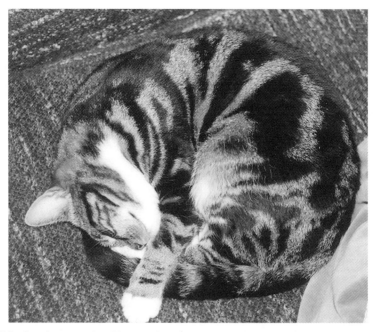

Fig. 10.1 Breed-associated problems are less common amongst cats, probably because of the continued popularity of the 'mog'. © Ann F. Stonehouse.

Conformation-induced or genetic?

Breed-related problems in domestic pets are often broadly divided into two overlapping categories: conformation-induced and genetic. Conformation-induced problems are the result of breeding for a particular physical characteristic such as gait, hip angle, face shape, or eye shape and size. The malocclusion from the foreshortened upper jaw and undershot lower jaw of the Boxer, for example, contributes to dental disease; the facial skin folds and drooping eyes of the Bloodhound increase the risk of skin-fold dermatitis and chronic conjunctivitis. Naturally, conformation-induced problems include a genetic component and should really come under the heading of polygenic defects (see later).

Genetic diseases are those that unexpectedly arise as a result of unfortunate breeding practices. In the search for breed characteristics and the 'perfect' animal, breeders sometimes resort to techniques that result in the expression of previously unsuspected and usually undesirable traits. These defects may include the expression of mutated genes and can have significant biomedical consequences. Manx cats, for example, are a tail-less breed arising from a gene mutation, but linked to the gene for tail-lessness is a mortality gene which results in the death, at or around birth, of a percentage of every litter from a pure mating. Inherited abnormalities in cats are less well recognised than in dogs so this chapter will concentrate on the dog diseases.

Diseases that are inherited or have a major genetic component are extremely important in companion animal practice. There are over 300 recognised inherited disease entities and this number is increasing rapidly. Many of these genetic conditions serve as models for human genetic diseases and are valuable as research models.

A combination of certain breeding practices affects the frequency of occurrence of inherited defects. These practices include line-breeding, in-breeding, 'popular sire effect' where a champion show dog is extensively used at stud, and the maintenance of purebred dogs within isolated breed pools. An inherited basis for a disease is suspected where there is breed predisposition for the disease and where it occurs most frequently in certain breeding lines (see Table 10.1).

Type*	Explanation	Expression	Eradication	Comments
Autosomal dominant	Gene is present on an autosome and only one copy of gene need be mutated to produce disease	Autosomal diseases pass directly from one generation to the next	Relatively easy *if dominant gene is fully expressed*	Difficult to identify mode of inheritance of partially penetrant characteristics
Autosomal recessive	Homozygous for expression: heterozygous are carriers	May skip generations: needs mating of two carriers	Identification of carriers crucial	Commonest mode of inheritance of single gene traits
X-linked recessive	Genes for disease on X chromosome: females carriers	Disease expressed in affected males, rarely in homozygous females	Identify female carriers	e.g. haemophilia A and B
Sex-limited inheritance	Genes carried by both sexes	Disease only expressed in one sex	Identify carriers	e.g. cryptorchidism
Polygenic defects	More than one gene locus influences expression of certain defects	Environment probably plays an important role in expression	Very difficult	e.g. hip dysplasia

* Mendelian genetics: dogs have 78 chromosomes (38 pairs of autosomes and two sex chromosomes).

Table 10.1   Modes of inheritance*.

The *expression* of an inherited disease results from and is more or less affected by the interaction of the genetic status of the animal with environmental factors. This results, in some cases, in a significant variation in features such as age of onset, rate of progression or severity. Examples of such environmentally affected diseases include hip dysplasia in large breeds and familial nephropathy in a range of breeds.

Naturally, conformation-induced problems have a genetic component. The difficulty lies in deciding when a conformation-induced problem is sufficiently serious to warrant doing something about it. For example, Springer Spaniels have a tendency to suffer chronic, recurrent otitis externa related to having heavy pinnae that effectively close the ear canal. The drooping ears are characteristic of the breed and are supposed to serve a protective function for the eardrum by muffling the effect of the sound of gunshot, and for the ear canal by stopping entrance of foreign bodies during forays into the undergrowth.

However, how many dogs in the total Springer population actually suffer from otitis? The different categories of people who have contact with the breed will have different impressions of the incidence and seriousness of the problem. The spaniel owner with a chronically ill animal feels the full effect of disease; similarly, the clinical veterinarian, exposed mostly to the unhealthy animals, may also feel there is a high incidence of problem within the breed. On the other hand, the show judge who sees the best and healthiest specimens may only acknowledge the soundness of the breed, and the breeder may choose to turn a blind eye to the problem, or not appreciate its significance in the overall health and performance of the breed. Also, what role do the following factors play in the incidence of otitis externa:

- breed conformation;
- environmental factors such as frequent wetting of the ear;
- breed tendency to seborrhoea;
- breed tendency to a compromised immune system that diminishes resistance to ear infection?

As in most other limited populations, detrimental genes and hereditary defects may accumulate. To some extent this is the price to be paid for the diversity of the breeds. This is where the research veterinarian and geneticist come in. It is only when statistical evaluation of a particular disease entity within a breed is available that those concerned are in a position actively to improve the breed. By developing and using appropriate screening tests for those defects known to be hereditary, and using that information when selecting breeding stock, the prevalence of these defects can be kept under control even if they are not completely eradicated.

Current screening tests

Modes of inheritance can be complicated, and some diseases only become apparent later in an animal's life, perhaps after it has already bred. Different screening methods for the recognition of affected and carrier animals are needed.

Clinical screening can be used in some diseases such as hip and elbow dysplasia, and some of the eye diseases. In these cases, specially trained veterinarians examine animals clinically, analyse test results, and give the animals a score based on clearly defined parameters. Depending on score results, the animal is then passed or failed as fit for breeding. With some of the eye diseases this examination may be done as early as 6–12 weeks old; with the skeletal problems, radiographs are usually taken at 12–18 months.

However, not all hereditary diseases can be detected and eliminated by clinical screening alone. In some cases, clinically normal dogs can be carriers of disease which will affect future generations. DNA testing using blood samples or cheek swabs from puppies is an exciting and accurate tool for identifying carriers so that they can be excluded from a breeding programme at an early stage. Two such screening tests are currently available – for progressive retinal atrophy in Irish Setters, and copper toxicosis in Bedlington Terriers – and more are being developed.

For future tests to be effective, certain issues need to be addressed, such as whether testing should be voluntary or compulsory, and whether results should be publically available, but genetic screening offers tremendous potential for identifying inherited conditions.

So, who is responsible?

There are four categories of people who have an influence on the breeding of dogs and cats:
- pet-owners;
- show judges;
- veterinarians and geneticists;
- breeders.

Pet-owners

Pet-owners experience the worry and expense of owning an unhealthy pet. They purchase their pet in good faith, but often with little knowledge of the breed risk for disease, and may have to suffer severe consequences including early euthanasia of the pet on the grounds of unsuitable temperament or physical disease; common examples of this include Cavalier King Charles Spaniels with early heart disease, Flat-coated Retrievers with malignant tumours in middle age, West Highland Terriers with chronic skin disease (Fig. 10.2), or Bernese Mountain dogs crippled by hip and elbow dysplasia. As breeders often keep the best of the litter themselves, there is also an increased risk that unwitting owners buy a second-rate pet in terms of health.

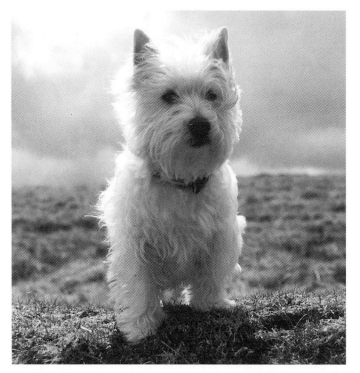

Fig. 10.2 Skin problems in West Highland White Terriers are an example of the increasing incidence of breed-associated health problems. © Ann F. Stonehouse.

Judges

Show judges see the best individuals within a breed. Although usually experienced breeders themselves, this may affect their assessment of the seriousness of a problem within a breed. Judges have considerable power to influence breeding activities through demanding or condemning more extreme breed traits. It is therefore important that they are made to appreciate the health significance of a particular problem through inclusion in all breed-improvement discussions, as they are a crucial group in helping to improve breed health.

Veterinarians

These can be divided into three categories:
- The clinical veterinarian who works at the level of the individual and most often sees only the unhealthy results of intensive breeding. He treats the affected animal, and can make general breeding recommendations. He may have some influence with breeders at a local level.

- The veterinarian with a serious interest in cat and dog breeding can develop a deeper relationship with a range of breeders, and actively work with them to improve their breeds through selection based on scientific data as well as knowledge of appearance, conformation, performance and so on. Often these veterinarians are breeders themselves, and serve as the link between the veterinary profession and the committed breeder. They work at a national level.
- The specialist veterinarian at the university or teaching institution works with the geneticist and research scientist to provide the scientific and statistical evidence for routes and means of inheritable disease transmission, and to develop appropriate screening tests. He often provides the expertise necessary for clinical or biochemical diagnosis of disease. Information is disseminated and shared with veterinarians and breed societies at an international level.

The ugly Golden Retriever bitch I described in Chapter 8 serves as an example of the different levels at which veterinarians work. In my professional opinion as a clinical veterinarian with a working knowledge of the breed I would not recommend her for breeding based on her undistinguished appearance. Of course, appearance is not everything: temperament and performance are equally if not more important.

The breeder-veterinarian might well have decided that the presence of excellent temperament justified her use in breeding, but would advise carefully matching her with a sound dog that would enhance her strengths and diminish her weaknesses. Through his intimate knowledge of the breed or through working closely with reputable breeders he might be more concerned about the incidence of hip dysplasia in her family line.

The investigatory veterinarian at the university working with geneticists would score the hip radiographs and provide the evidence for the familial tendency to hip dysplasia which would affect the decision to breed from the bitch or not.

Breeders

Breeders ultimately control the whole situation. They, also, can be subdivided into several categories. Most serious breeders care deeply about the health and welfare of their animals, who represent status and income as well as being affectionate and rewarding companions. These breeders are very dedicated in their search to maintain and improve a breed, and have a deep knowledge of the breed, especially their own breeding lines. Problems arise when these breeders are pressurised by unfortunate descriptions of breed standards as well as misinterpretation of these standards by show judges to produce exaggerated anatomical features that adversely affect the health and well-being of individuals.

The enthusiastic amateur breeder includes the interested pet-owner. Although well-meaning, their desire to have 'just one litter' or to 'have a go' at breeding can result in sub-standard animals through breeding from second-rate or incompatible stock. For example, someone with a German Shepherd bitch may not know that she should have her pet's hips assessed for hip dysplasia before mating with the neighbour's fine and seemingly sound German Shepherd dog. The resulting litter might have a high incidence of hip dysplasia.

It can be very difficult for a pet-owner looking for a new puppy or kitten to differentiate the serious committed breeder from the enthusiastic but misguided amateur, or the downright cheat. All can be very convincing in their stories.

A friend had the interesting experience recently of seeking a Staffordshire Bull Terrier puppy as a companion and eventual replacement for her old 'Staffie'. The first breeder she contacted tried to sell her an unsocialised, unfriendly bitch aged 16 weeks with an inguinal hernia, undershot jaw and flop ear (Staffies' ears should be neatly folded). The bitch was also recovering from ringworm. He assured her that in a couple of weeks the puppy would be perfectly friendly and socialised, the hernia was simply an accident at birth (although the mother also had a hernia), and that the ear would reform with massage. He was asking half the normal price for the bitch on the condition he could have two litters from her. Neither the dog nor bitch who were parents to the litter were good examples of the breed standard although nice dogs in themselves. The breeder also admitted that some of his dogs' progeny were used for illegal fighting.

The second breeder my friend approached had bred and shown top champions. Her puppies were fully socialised and were sold vaccinated, wormed, ear marked and with the commitment that they would be hip and elbow radiographed at one year (although dysplasia is not a problem in the breed, there have been a handful of cases reported). The contrast between the quality of the puppies, and the level of care in breeding and raising them, was very marked — and she has been delighted with the dog puppy she purchased from this breeder.

Unscrupulous breeders produce animals for personal gain and have no fundamental interest in their health or welfare. This group includes the owners of puppy farms and pet-owners who allow their pet to breed indiscriminately or who deliberately seek to enhance negative characteristics such as aggression. This is the most difficult subgroup with which to work.

Control of inherited disease

The combined efforts of veterinarians, breeders and geneticists can make a significant difference to the number and severity of hereditary diseases affecting dogs, but success requires education, communication and co-operation between all the parties involved. There are several stages involved in working to reduce or eradicate an inheritable disease:

1 Breeders must accept that there is a problem with their animals. This may be difficult: it has been likened to admitting your child is an idiot.
2 Schemes need accurate diagnosis of the disease phenotype, ideally before sexual maturity, and knowledge of the mode of inheritance and the

magnitude of the problem in both the general population and the affected subpopulation.

3 This information should be presented to the breeders through their breed clubs by veterinarians, and advice offered about altering breeding policies. For example, if a particular gene was found to be carried by a favoured stud dog, that dog would have to be eliminated from the breeding population.

4 The new breeding policies should be monitored to ensure that they are having the desired effect. Problems sometimes arise when selective breeding aimed at controlling one condition leads to increased prevalence of another.

Swedish canine genetic health programmes

Sweden has provided a model for success with its canine genetic health programmes which are administered by the Swedish Kennel Club. Screening and eradication programmes for hip dysplasia and hereditary eye disease have been in place for the last thirty years; more recently formal programmes for elbow arthroses, haemophilia A, progressive nephropathy and canine leukocyte adhesion deficiency have been added. New genetic health programmes for chronic valvular disease in Cavalier King Charles Spaniels and patellar luxation in Finnish Spitzes have been developed. Analysis of the earliest programmes has shown them to be effective both in reducing the incidence of disease and in terms of cost-effectiveness.

For example, the hip dysplasia scheme has been running since 1958, and administered by the Kennel Club since 1970. It serves as a model for other genetic health programmes mentioned above. Between 1976 and 1989 the prevalence of hip dysplasia decreased dramatically in a number of breeds. In a paper by Swenson et al (1997b) the authors describe why the Swedish hip dysplasia scheme is particularly successful. Important factors for success include:

- A tradition of good cooperation and knowledge-sharing between veterinarians, the Swedish Kennel Club, breeders and geneticists.
- Over 80% of dogs are purebred and registered with one single body, the Swedish Kennel Club.
- There are few stray dogs, and dogs in general are well cared for.
- Registration by tattooing or micro-chipping is mandatory before entering any of the screening programmes.
- There is central evaluation of radiographs for hip dysplasia using a score of 1–4 (slight–severe dysplasia) by one radiologist who has examined over 83 000 radiographs from seven different breeds.
- Owners a sign an agreement that the results of the evaluation are registered by the Swedish Kennel Club, and this information is available to the public.
- Since 1983 as a service to breeders, it has been possible to obtain information on the coxofemoral joint status of any individual dog for which radiographs have been evaluated, all the progeny of any individual dog, all dogs within a breed in relation to year of birth, and all breeding dogs in relation to year of birth and litters born.

• Since 1984 it has been mandatory that the coxofemoral joint status be known for the sire and the dam if the progeny are to be registered by the Swedish Kennel Club.

In addition, an inventory has been compiled on the presence, prevalence and ranked severity (for the individual, and the population of each breed) of known hereditary defects. The purpose is to gather information on the actual situation within each breed for both well defined and documented conditions, and for what is known by the breeders but not necessarily by the veterinarians.

Efforts are being made to inform and educate dog show judges about the health risks associated with selecting for exaggerated anatomical features. A video for this purpose has been produced in collaboration with Australian veterinarian and international show judge, Dr Harold Spira; it contains slides and motion pictures of the extreme variables and what to strive towards in improving soundness in different breeds.

Figures for cost-effectiveness of the current schemes also support their effectiveness in reducing genetic disease.

Conclusion

Persuading breeders to admit to a problem with their animals is only the first stage in establishing a genetic health programme. Effective health policies then require dialogue and cooperation between breed societies and veterinarians at local, national and international level, and with geneticists.

The clinical veterinarian can advise potential owners about the health risks associated with certain breeds, the husbandry factors that may affect expression of disease, and the importance of making an informed decision about breeding. This information should be part of both pre-selection and puppy/kitten care programmes.

With thanks to Åke Hedhammar for proof-reading and comments.

References and further reading

Hedhammar, Å. (1995). Breeding healthier dogs in Sweden. AKC Parent Club Genetics Conference, Hamilton Park Conference Center, New Jersey.

Hedhammar, Å., Häggström, J., Håkanson, B.W., Swenson, L., Audell, L. and Darell, A-M. (1996). Canine genetic health programs by the Swedish Kennel Club – evaluated, developed and extended. *Svensk Veterinärtidning* **48**(8–9), 395–401 (Swedish, English summary).

Petersen-Jones, S.M. (1996). The problem of inherited diseases: do we have the answers? *Journal of Small Animal Practice* 299–302.

Swenson, L., Audell, L. and Hedhammar, Å. (1997a). Prevalence and inheritance of and selection for elbow arthroses in Bernese Mountain dogs and Rottweilers in Sweden and benefit/cost analysis of a screening and control programme. *Journal of the American Veterinary Medical Association* **210**(2), 1–7.

Swenson, L., Audell, L. and Hedhammar, Å. (1997b). Prevalence and inheritance of and selection for hip dysplasia in seven breeds of dogs in Sweden and benefit:cost analysis of a screening and control programme. *Journal of the American Veterinary Medical Association* **210**(2), 207–214.

Wills, J. and Wolf, A. (eds) (1993). *Handbook of Feline Medicine*. Pergamon Press, Oxford.

The Influence of Environmental Factors on Health

11

David H. Lloyd

Introduction

The influence of environment on animal health is often dismissed. The familiarity of the home, the workplace, and the streets or fields where we live tends to make us assume that these areas present little risk (Fig. 11.1). Where potential hazards are recognised we commonly avoid taking action on the basis that environmental factors cannot readily be controlled. Often the risks are difficult to evaluate, and thus the benefit of taking action cannot be assessed or appreciated.

Nevertheless, the environment has always presented substantial health risks to both man and animals. Lack of hygiene and poor understanding of the pathogenesis of disease have led to some notable pandemics in the past. In Europe, the Black Death raged through the continent during the fourteenth century and resulted in the death of about 25% of the population. Renamed 'the Plague' it killed 70 000 people in London alone in the year 1664–65. The disease, caused by infection with the bacterium *Yersinia pestis*, carried by the black rat, was principally transmitted and inoculated into its victims by the rat flea, *Xenopsylla cheopis*.

In our modern society we are protected from many of the environmental problems of the past. State hygiene regulations, the use of disinfectants and

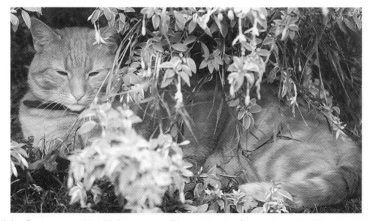

Fig. 11.1 Environmental health factors are of increasing significance in pet health and may be the most difficult group to manage. © Ann F. Stonehouse.

detergents in the home, and the availability of powerful drugs to cure disease have made us rather complacent. Even so, limited but sometimes serious outbreaks of disease remind us that the environment can still present significant risks. Deaths in man associated with contamination of meat by *Escherichia coli* O147 in Scotland provide a recent example. Furthermore, the very chemicals which we use to protect ourselves and our animals can constitute an additional hazard.

In this chapter various environmental factors which are involved directly or indirectly in animal disease will be described with the aim of raising consciousness of the challenges present in the home and elsewhere. An approach to client information aimed at promoting the concept of health maintenance as opposed to the treatment of disease is also outlined.

Climatic factors

Sun exposure, and both high and low temperature and humidity, are risk factors which are often ignored in relation to pets even when owners take precautions themselves.

Ultraviolet light

Damage to the skin by the sun's rays is caused principally by ultraviolet light, which is conventionally divided into UVA (320–400 nm), UVB (290–320 nm) and UVC (100–290 nm). UVA levels are fairly constant during the day: exposure is associated with tanning and, in the long term, with dermal connective tissue damage. UVA contributes little to erythema and burning but can augment the carcinogenic effects of UVB.

UVB transmits much greater electromagnetic energy and is the principal agent responsible for sunburn, suntanning and cutaneous neoplasia. It is most intense during the middle of the day, but, unlike UVA, is absorbed by window glass. UVC is absorbed almost completely by ozone in the atmosphere and stratosphere (Ananthaswamy and Kripke, 1991; Habif, 1996). Ultraviolet intensity is elevated at high altitudes, and exposure is increased in highly reflective environments such as white sand and snow. Chemical sunscreens can block UVB but are less effective against UVA unless specifically balanced to block UVA as well. Because UVB-blocking suncreens inhibit pigmentation responses generated by UVB they increase the effect of exposure to UVA.

Unpigmented skin is readily damaged if exposed to sunlight, even in the temperate zones. Acute skin damage, which occurs in sunburn and photosensitisation, needs to be differentiated from more chronic effects which may lead to the formation of actinic keratoses or tumours including squamous cell carcinoma and basal cell tumours (Gilchrist, 1995; Scott et al 1995). Chronic dermal damage, which leads to solar elastosis in man, may also affect dogs and cats.

In recent years there has been an increasing realisation that one of the significant effects of ultraviolet-induced cutaneous damage is immunosuppression. This appears to be mediated via damage to dendritic antigen-presenting cells, including the epidermal Langerhans cells, and also through the actions of suppressor T lymphocytes (Ananthaswamy and Kripke, 1991; Vink et al, 1996). The effects can be both local and systemic and may operate at cutaneous sites distant from the point of exposure. They impair immune rejection of tumours, allergic responses and immunity to micro-organisms (Ananthaswamy and Kripke, 1991; Yager and Wilcock, 1994; Vink et al, 1996). Reduction of immunity to viruses associated with exposure to sunlight may also be involved in the pathogenesis of some cutaneous tumours with viral aetiology, although evidence for this in dogs and cats is lacking. Exposure of animals and man to the harmful effects of ultraviolet light is steadily increasing because of the effects of stratospheric ozone depletion. Estimates of global ozone trends indicate that this depletion affects the whole world but there appears to be an accelerated rate of ozone loss at higher latitudes, including Europe and North America. Unfortunately, this elevation in ultraviolet penetration is concentrated in the highly damaging UVB region (Ananthaswamy and Kripke, 1991).

Actinic damage in dogs and cats can occur at any unpigmented skin sites, including areas of depigmentation or scarring, that are not protected by the coat. Less protection is offered by thin or unpigmented pelage. Solar dermatitis is a phototoxic reaction to sun exposure in which the severity is related to the duration and intensity of the incident ultraviolet light, and in chronic lesions to the frequency of exposure (Scott et al, 1995). In dogs, the lesions most commonly affect the unpigmented skin of the nose or muzzle (canine nasal solar dermatitis) but can involve the abdomen and flanks in animals that sunbathe in lateral recumbency, or the entire ventral skin if they are held on or above reflective concrete surfaces (Scott et al, 1995). Short-term exposure leads to erythema and scaling which affects white or lightly pigmented areas. Subsequently there is exudation and crusting and, in severe cases, ulceration. Scarring occurs with loss of hair in adjacent areas of skin following severe damage. Exposure over several seasons leads to more extensive lesions with skin thickening, formation of comedones and follicular cysts, folliculitis and furunculosis. Necrosis and fistulation may occur. Ultimately squamous cell carcinoma, haemangioma or haemangio-sarcoma are likely sequelae (Rosencrantz, 1993). The disease in cats follows a similar progression and affects particularly the tips of the ears in white cats, but may affect any unpigmented area including the lips and eyelid margins (Rosencrantz, 1993). The course is often chronic.

Diagnosis is based on the clinical signs and history of sun exposure supported by histopathology. Phototoxic reactions need to be differentiated from photosensitivity which, though not common, has been reported in the dog (Hudson and Florax, 1991). Photosensitivity reactions may be differentiated clinically by their severity, which is not dependent on prolonged or intense sun exposure. In early cases avoidance or protection from the sun will lead to resolution of the lesions. Water-resistant sun blocking agents (UVA and UVB) are helpful and clothing designed to cover the vulnerable areas may also be used. More severe lesions may need to be treated with topical corticosteroids and, if infected, with antibiotics. Where neoplastic or precancerous changes are present specific therapy for these conditions should be instituted.

Although owners are often aware of the risks of ultraviolet light to human skin they seldom take account of the effects of exposure to their pets. The long-term nature of many of the effects of exposure to ultraviolet light and the increasing intensity of exposure at the earth's surface mean that we should expect to see a growing range of problems in dogs and cats which are exposed to the sun.

Temperature and humidity

The effects of environmental temperature and humidity are more difficult to quantify. Excessive heat, particularly in dogs which are exercising and do not have access to water (Assia et al, 1989) or who are locked in over-heated cars in summer, can induce heat stroke. Icy conditions may cause frost bite, particularly at the extremities and in animals with circulatory problems. Away from the extremes, the effects are more gradual but heat stress and exhaustion may still be significant.

Although dogs and cats do not rely on sweating to control their body temperature, heat exchange via the skin is important, and animals with long and dense coats are at much greater risk. Coat and skin colour may also be important factors. Dark skin absorbs heat in hot and sunny weather whereas glossy, light coloured coats are protective (Scott, 1990).

There is a widely held but erroneous belief that dogs and cats do not possess sweat glands. In fact sweat glands are abundant over the body surface. On the hairy skin nearly all of these are epitrichial, i.e. associated with the hair follicles. Atrichial sweat glands are found on hairless skin, particularly on the footpads in dogs and cats; they are occasionally present also in hairy areas (Jenkinson, 1990). Both types of gland respond to adrenaline in dogs and cats, and increased sweating occurs when they are excited or subjected to stress. The role of sweat is principally protective in these species, including the maintenance of hydration, flexibility and resistance to friction in the stratum corneum (Jenkinson, 1990). The humidity at the skin surface and within the coat adjacent to the skin is strongly influenced by sweating. Production of sebum by the sebaceous glands, to form a film at the skin surface, is also important in maintaining surface flexibility and the humidity of the stratum corneum.

The influence of sweat and sebum on skin surface humidity is modulated by coat density and length. The effects of ambient temperature and humidity and of incident radiation (from the sun, radiators and fires in the home) are in turn influenced by the structure of the coat, occlusion (e.g. skin folds, tail, axilla), the effects of wind, and behavioural responses by the dog or cat. Behavioural options are, of course, dependent on the environments made accessible to the animal by the owner.

The skin microenvironment

Little work has been done on the microenvironment of the skin of dogs and cats. However, Chesney (1993) reviewed aspects of water balance on the skin and has demonstrated that variations in skin hydration exist at different sites over the canine skin surface and that scaly skin is drier than normal skin (Chesney, 1995). Comparing relative humidity over the skin surface in Newfoundland dogs he showed that the level was substantially higher on occluded areas, beneath the tail and under the neck (c. 70%), compared with sites on the rump, thigh and chest (c. 50%) (Chesney, 1996). However, when he compared the non-lesional skin of normal and atopic dogs, he was unable to demonstrate differences (Chesney, 1995).

Skin surface humidity and temperature are of great importance in determining the nature and population density of the skin microflora. Changes in skin surface conditions may allow the establishment of pathogens, promoting the onset of bacterial and fungal disease (Lloyd, 1980; McBride, 1993). It is well recognised that skin infections are more prevalent in hot, humid conditions. Temperature is of more importance in animals with thermoregulatory sweating (Lloyd, 1980) in which increased humidity is a consequence of elevated ambient temperature. The situation in dogs and cats has not been studied but it has been postulated that the elevated frequency of infection in dogs in areas such as the ventral neck and beneath the tail may be associated with higher humidity (Chesney, 1996). Changes in the surface microenvironment of the skin may also be induced by changes in peripheral blood flow and in the permeability of the epidermis associated with haemodynamic control mechanisms, stress factors, and inflammatory changes associated with both local and systemic disease (Mason and Lloyd, 1990, 1996; Scheuplein, 1991).

Chemicals in the environment

Noxious chemicals in the external environment, in the home and at the workplace, are also a significant risk factor to dogs and cats. Poisoning may occur as a result of ingestion or absorption via the skin, or the reaction may be restricted to the skin and manifested as a contact reaction. Longer-term irritant effects of chemicals in contact with the skin or absorbed systemically may predispose to neoplasia. Studies in the United States have shown that topical insecticides used for flea control may pose an increased risk of bladder cancer. The risk was related to frequency of use and was substantially greater when insecticides were applied more than twice per year. This risk was enhanced in obese dogs (Glickman et al, 1989).

Contact dermatitis

The skin reaction to noxious chemicals can be a direct irritant effect or may, after repeated exposure, lead to hypersensitivity classically involving a delayed, type IV response. Severe, acute irritant reactions result from contact with strong acids and alkalis or preservatives such as creosote. More commonly the reactions are caused by prolonged or repeated contact with the causative agent which may initially have mild and inapparent effects. Modes of exposure can be deceptive and unexpected in the complex home environment or at the owner's workplace, where many different chemicals may be routinely used for washing, disinfecting, deodorising, controlling pests, or as lubricants or by-products in industrial processes. An example of unexpected contact irritation is the effect of disinfectant left wet on a treated floor. The concentration applied is safe but concentration of droplets caused by evaporation may then lead to damaging residual amounts which can cause skin irritation when the animal lies on the supposedly clean surface.

Hypersensitivity reactions to a wide variety of agents have been reported but these are rarely well documented. There is good evidence of hypersensitivity to a number of plants (*Tradescantia fluminensis, Hippeastrum* leaves and bulbs, Asian jasmine and dandelion leaves) and to synthetic textiles (Scott et al, 1995). The lesions induced depend on the nature of the causative agent and the level of exposure. Solid agents cause lesions on exposed and relatively hairless skin which do not extend into the hairy areas, whereas liquids can cause lesions at any point on the skin. The lesions are typically pruritic, maculopapular rashes but vesicle formation may occur and, in chronic exposure, alopecia, hyperpigmentation and lichenification may be seen. With severe pruritus, excoriation and acute moist dermatitis may occur.

Histopathological examination of biopsy specimens cannot be used to differentiate contact irritation and hypersensitivity (Yager and Wilcock, 1994). Diagnosis is therefore based on the history of contact with the causative agent and then exclusion from it, or on provocative exposure or patch testing. Irritant agents often affect several individuals in a group of animals, whereas this is uncommon in contact hypersensitivity. Resolution of lesions occurs soon after contact with the offending substance is prevented but topical or systemic glucocorticoids may be required to control irritation; long-term therapy is required in cases where contact with the agent cannot be eliminated. It should be noted that contact hypersensitivity is a rare disease in dogs and cats and is greatly overdiagnosed.

Recurrent injury caused by other environmental factors may cause lesions which simulate contact irritation. It is important to investigate fully the animal's interaction with its environment in order to identify such causes. Dr David Grant has described a case of a cat which developed hair loss, erythema and skin thickening over the neck which was caused by the heat of a radiator situated just above its feeding bowl (Grant, personal communication).

Atmospheric pollution

Chemicals and particulate matter in the atmosphere may also pose risks to pets. Air quality in cities and industrial areas can be severely downgraded when temperature inversions trap pollutants from vehicles and factories. Polluted city air can contain substantial amounts of noxious gases, including oxides of nitrogen, sulphur dioxide, carbon monoxide and ozone, and can lead to cardiac and respiratory problems, including hypoxia, in man and animals. Concentrations of these gases are highest in cities, particularly near roads, with the exception of ozone which tends to be in higher concentration in city suburbs, open spaces in cities and in rural areas. Chronic hypoxia has been associated with the occurrence of neoplasia affecting the chemoreceptors of the aortic and carotid bodies in dogs (Hayes, 1975). The frequency of lung cancer in dogs and cats has increased at least twofold during the last 20 years (Moulton, 1990) and this may also be associated with city living. Russian data indicate that dogs in cities have a higher incidence of lung cancer than those in the country (Leake, 1961).

The atmosphere is generally much less polluted in rural areas but animals may suffer from acute exposure to agricultural chemicals, particularly pesticides, at certain times of the year. Pollens and mould spores also cause allergic reactions in hypersensitive animals that may be associated with upper respiratory tract disease or may lead to allergic skin reactions (Sture et al, 1995).

In the home, tobacco smoke is a potential hazard; it may be associated with a risk of lung cancer in dogs and with respiratory disease in the cat. In dogs, the risk posed by smoke appears to be related to skull shape and is greater for animals with shorter or medium length noses (Reif et al, 1992).

House dust

House dust, and particularly the presence of house dust mites, is also a significant risk factor for skin and respiratory disease in dogs and cats. Allergy to species of *Dermatophagoides* is the most common cause of atopy among dogs in Europe (Sture et al, 1995). Problems are exacerbated in houses with poor hygiene, and measures aimed at reducing mite populations are often beneficial. Both inhalation and skin absorption of allergen are factors in this disease: the fact that the pets spend most of their time at carpet level means that they are in a zone of high exposure.

Infections and infestations

Ectoparasites

Ectoparasitic infestations are the most common problems encountered in small animal practice. Amongst these, flea infestation is the most important and is strongly influenced by the management procedures adopted by the owner and by the grooming activities of the animal. In the western world, *Ctenocephalides felis felis* is the most prevalent flea in almost every country (reviewed by Dryden and Rust, 1994) although *Ct. canis* has been reported to be more common in Austria, Ireland and New Zealand; the human flea, *Pulex irritans*, is sometimes found on dogs and cats in significant numbers. Moderate levels of flea infestation do not cause significant skin irritation in healthy animals although high levels can result in anaemia. However, if flea bite hypersensitivity exists then pruritic skin disease occurs, varying from a mild erythema to an extensive syndrome with crusted papules, scaling and alopecia. In mild cases, particularly in cats, the only signs may be overgrooming with slight ventral erythema and hair loss. This is often unnoticed by the owner. Fleas may not be readily found on animals with flea allergy and even careful veterinary examination may fail to reveal the presence of adult fleas or flea faeces. This may make it difficult to convince the house-proud owner that his or her house is infested with fleas and that rigorous flea control measures are necessary.

Successful elimination of fleas from the home environment necessitates an understanding of the biology of the flea (Dryden and Rust, 1994) and involves treatment both of the house itself and of the dogs and cats which are resident there. The environmental problem is caused first of all by flea eggs which are laid on the animal and fall off wherever the animal goes; they are concentrated in places where the animal jumps or shakes itself. The eggs give rise to larvae which are positively geotropic and negatively phototropic and thus move deep into the carpet or crevices in the floor, and into shaded areas. The area under the owner's bed is often highly infested. The larvae give rise to pupae which are formed within the carpet or in crevices and are thus protected from the action of sprays and fumigants. The pupae may remain dormant for many months until stimulated to emerge by the presence of animals.

Populations can be kept low by periodic treatment of animals with persistent insecticides, e.g. fipronil, by the use of insecticidal flea collars, by the use of systemic insecticides which kill fleas when they ingest the product in the blood, and by the use of hygienic measures such as rigorous vacuum cleaning. However, the environment continues to act as a reservoir of infestation unless treated effectively. In winter, when the external temperature remains below about 13°C, adult fleas are not present outside but during the rest of the year animals which leave the home will acquire fleas and the probability of bringing them into the home is high.

Frequent treatment of the home environment is needed to ensure that the adults are destroyed as they emerge from the pupae. Better long-term solutions are provided by products which remain active against the larvae in the environment for long periods of time, such as the insect growth regulators, e.g. methoprene or fenoxycarb, or sodium polyborate powder. The latter has the advantage that it also kills house dust mites. An alternative is the use of oral lufenuron, which is absorbed by female fleas when they feed on the blood of the host and passes into the eggs, leading to failure of hatching. However, long-term treatment of all animals entering the environment is needed before control can be achieved. Hence this product is not appropriate in severe flea allergy.

In animals with flea allergy it is important to prevent flea bites. A combination of a topical animal treatment, applied frequently enough to prevent biting and applied to all animals living in the house, and a long-term environmental product which prevents maturation of fleas in the home will be effective if the allergic animal does not visit other places where fleas are prevalent, e.g. houses of friends. Control may also fail if infested animals visit the house either by invitation (with the owner's friends) or via cat or dog flaps. Feral animals living close to the home may also enable the persistence of significant local environmental reservoirs of fleas and cause the flea control programme to fail.

Other ectoparasitic infestations (mites, lice, ticks) can be acquired during visits to other houses, to the park, or on walks in the country, either by contact with infested animals or from environmental sources. Some of these problems can be predicted. For example, veterinarians will be aware of areas of country in the region of their practices in which infestation with the harvest mite, *Neotrombicula autumnalis*, occurs every autumn. Similarly, holiday visits to tick-infested areas may lead to predictable infestations. Such problems can be dealt with as they occur but are better foreseen and prevented, either by avoidance of the infested regions or by prophylactic treatment. Persistent insecticides such as fipronil or permethrin applied prior to the period of risk may be effective.

In warmer climates arthropod-borne diseases such as leishmaniasis, ehrlichiosis, babesiosis and heartworm are significant hazards; owners need to be advised on precautionary measures to minimise the risk of infection. These diseases are a particular hazard for animals on holiday with owners from non-endemic regions who are commonly unaware of the risks.

Unexpected infestations may also occur when animals with inapparent infestations are introduced into a household. Infestations of young dogs with *Cheyletiella yasguri* can be very mild or subclinical but may be passed to other dogs which may display clinical disease. Stress factors associated with poor management or concurrent disease may also cause subclinical infestation to become clinically significant, again providing unexpected disease. The presence of the tapeworm, *Dipylidium caninum*, in dogs or cats is strong evidence for infestations with fleas or, on rare occasions, lice which act as the intermediate hosts.

Dermatophytosis

Dermatophytosis, caused by *Microsporum canis*, is another disease which is associated with environmental contamination or is acquired from clinically affected cats or dogs (Deboer and Moriello, 1995; Deboer et al, 1995). Cats are the principal reservoir host and feral cats commonly suffer from endemic disease, thus providing a continuing source of infection for pets. Adults, particularly long-haired cats, may remain chronically infected – sometimes with minimal clinical signs – or may act as carriers. Clinical disease, however, is most prevalent in kittens. Transmission from infected pets to the owner's family often occurs. The infective arthrospores are shed in large numbers and can survive for many months in the home environment (Sparkes et al, 1994). Treatment of infected cats and dogs, especially long-haired animals, can be a major challenge. A combination of clipping, long-term topical and systemic therapy, and vigorous environmental disinfection is required.

Other species of the genera *Microsporum* and *Trichophyton* also sporadically affect dogs and cats. The infections are generally acquired from the environment and are not readily transmitted between pets or to their owners. *M. gypseum* is a geophilic dermatophyte which is found in certain rural environments, and causes relatively frequent canine infections in those areas, but may be absent in other regions. Infection with *Trichophyton mentagrophytes* is also acquired from the environment.

The principal reservoir is in rodents: infection occurs particularly in dogs that are attracted to rural rodent habitats, such as Jack Russell Terriers. Treatment of these diseases is based on the use of systemic antifungal drugs such as griseofulvin and ketoconazole. Long-term therapy may be needed but contamination of the home is not usually a significant problem.

Where dogs or cats live in flats and never have access to the exterior it is much easier to control infections and infestations. However, even brief visits by other animals can readily introduce problems such as fleas or ringworm. Such transient visits may be forgotten by the owner and only identified by careful questioning by the clinician.

Risk reduction strategies

Persuading owners to adopt practices that protect their animals from environmental risk factors such as those outlined above is not easy. The broad range of hazards and the fact that few of them have immediate or readily recognisable effects make educating clients a long-term and potentially time-consuming process. Strategies need to be adopted to engage the enthusiasm of the owners and their pride in their pets without implying that their home environment is unhygienic or creating a sense of panic. The veterinary surgeon will need to learn about the home and exercise environments occupied by the pet(s) and to analyse the identifiable risk factors so that appropriate advice can be provided.

Flea control is a particularly apt example. Flea-related problems are probably the most common events that bring clients to the veterinary practice. Explaining the life-cycle of the flea to the client in such a way as to enable an effective control programme to be instituted is surprisingly difficult. It seems so obvious to the veterinarian but owners probably leave the practice confused or misinformed in most cases, and flea control programmes frequently fail as a result. Diagrams of the life-cycle, used whilst explaining the problem, and well-illustrated leaflets which the owner can take away provide the key.

All dogs and cats will be exposed to fleas at some time in their lives unless they live in flea-free regions of the world or are kept in apartments in isolation from other animals (no animal visitors allowed). Thus the need for flea control and the regular supply of the selected anti-flea products will provide an opportunity to discuss the home environment and identify other risks and problems which need to be addressed. The flea control visits can be combined or associated with the regular health check. Such repeated visits should enable the long-term aspects of the environmental health programme to be established, involving a continuing dialogue in which the owner can discuss his or her pet's health, and the processes of client education can develop as part of the practice wellness programme. In this way it may be possible to persuade the owners to adopt other risk avoidance strategies appropriate to their pets. These might include modified exercise programmes for dogs with restricted airways to avoid busy roads or, in the case of harvest mite infestation, avoidance of rural areas known to harbour mites in late summer or the use of a persistent surface insecticide which kills the mites when they attempt to feed. For owners taking their animals into areas with endemic tick or insect-borne diseases, the use of topical acaricides can be recommended and information on the diurnal patterns of insect vector activity given to enable them to minimise the risks of exposure. In such cases, post-holiday health checks are advisable.

The risks posed by environmental hazards represent an area of veterinary practice which is at present insufficiently understood and underexploited. Many of the problems outlined above will undoubtedly become a lot more severe in years to come. Addressing these hazards and developing an environmental health strategy is likely to become increasingly necessary. This should not be regarded as a problem but rather as an opportunity to focus on strengthening the client–practitioner relationship and building a more effective approach to health amongst the veterinary community.

References

Ananthaswamy, H.N. and Kripke, M.L. (1991). Experimental skin carcinogenesis by ultraviolet radiation. In: Soter, N.A. and Baden, H.P. (eds). *Pathophysiology of Dermatologic Diseases*, (2nd edn). McGraw-Hill, New York, p 483–505.

Assia, E., Epstein, Y., Magazanik, A., Shapiro, Y. and Sohar, E. (1989). Plasma-cortisol levels in experimental heatstroke in dogs. *International Journal of Biometeorology* **33**, 85–88.

Catanzaro, T.E. (1998) *Building the Successful Veterinary Practice: Programs & Procedures* (Vol. 2). Iowa State University Press, Ames, Iowa.

Chesney, C.J. (1993). Water: its form, function and importance in the skin of domestic animals. *Journal of Small Animal Practice* **34**, 65–71.

Chesney, C.J. (1995). Measurement of skin hydration in normal dogs and in dogs with atopy or a scaling dermatosis. *Journal of Small Animal Practice* **36**, 305–309.

Chesney, C.J. (1996). Mapping the canine skin: a study of coat relative humidity in Newfoundland dogs. *Veterinary Dermatology* **7**, 35–41.

Deboer, D.J. and Moriello, K.A. (1995). Clinical update on feline dermatophytosis. Part I. *Compendium on Continuing Education* **17**(10), 1197–1203.

Deboer, D.L., Moriello, K.A. and Caurns, R. (1995). Clinical update on feline dermatophytosis. Part II. *Compendium on Continuing Education* **17** (12), 1471–1480.

Dryden, M. and Rust, M. (1994). The cat flea, biology, ecology and control. *Veterinary Parasitology* **52**, 1–19.

Gilchrist, B.A. (1995). *Photodamage*. Blackwell Science, Cambridge, U.K.

Glickman, L.T., Schofer, F.S., McKee, L.J., Reif, J.S. and Goldschmidt, M.H. (1989). Epidemiologic study of insecticide exposure, obesity, and risk of bladder cancer in household dogs. *Journal of Toxicology and Environmental Health* **28**, 407–414.

Habif, T.P. (1996). *Clinical Dermatology* (3rd edn). Mosby, St Louis, p 597–626, 649–720.

Hayes, H.H. (1975). An hypothesis for the aetiology of canine chemoreceptor system neoplasms, based on an epidemiological study of 73 cases among hospital patients. *Journal of Small Animal Practice* **16**, 337–343.

Hudson, W.E. and Florax, M.J.H. (1991). Photosensitization in foxhounds. *Veterinary Record* **128**, 618.

Jenkinson, D. McE. (1990). Sweat and sebaceous glands and their function in domestic animals. In: von Tscharner, C. and Halliwell, R.E.W. (eds) *Advances in Veterinary Dermatology. Volume 1.* Baillière Tindall, London, p 229–251.

Leake, C.D. (1961). Lung cancer in dogs. *Journal of the American Veterinary Medical Association* **173**, 85–86.

Lloyd, D.H. (1980). The inhabitants of the mammalian skin surface. *Proceedings of the Royal Society of Edinburgh* **79B**, 25–42.

McBride, M.E. (1993). Physical factors affecting the skin flora and skin disease. In: Noble, W.C. (ed) *The Skin Flora and Microbial Skin Disease.* Cambridge University Press, Cambridge, p 73–101.

Mason, I.S. and Lloyd, D. H. (1990). Factors influencing the penetration of bacterial antigens through canine skin. In: von Tscharner, C. and Halliwell, R.E.W. (eds) *Advances in Veterinary Dermatology. Volume 1.* Baillière Tindall, London, p 370–374.

Mason, I.S. and Lloyd, D.H. (1996) Evaluation of compound 48/80 as a model of immediate hypersensitivity in the skin of dogs. *Veterinary Dermatology* **7**, 81–83.

Moulton, J.E. (1990). *Tumors in Domestic Animals* (3rd edn). University of California Press, Berkley.

Reif, J.S., Dunn, K. ,Ogilvie, G.K. and Harris, C.K. (1992). Passive smoking and canine lung cancer risk. *American Journal of Epidemiology* **135**, 234–239.

Rosencrantz, W.S. (1993). Solar dermatitis. In: Griffin, C.E., Kwochka, K. W. and MacDonald, J.M. (eds) *Current Veterinary Dermatology. The Science and Art of Therapy.* Mosby Year Book, St Louis, p 302–315.

Scheuplein, R.J. (1991). Temperature regulation in the skin. In: Soter, N.A. and Baden, H.P. (eds) *Pathophysiology of Dermatologic Disease.* McGraw-Hill, New York, p 67–82.

Scott, D.W. (1980) Feline dermatology 1900–1978: a monograph. *Journal of the American Animal Hospital Association* **16**, 331.

Scott, D.W. (1990). The biology of hair growth and its disturbances. In: von Tscharner, C. and Halliwell, R.E.W. (eds) *Advances in Veterinary Dermatology. Volume 1.* Baillière Tindall, London, p 3–33.

Scott, D.W., Miller, W.H. and Griffin, C.E. (1995). *Muller and Kirk's Small Animal Dermatology* (5th edn). W.B. Saunders, Philadelphia.

Sparkes, A.H., Werrett, G., Stokes, C.R. and Gruffydd-Jones, T.J. (1994). *Microsporum canis:* inapparent carriage by cats and the viability of arthrospores. *Journal of Small Animal Practice* **35**, 397–401.

Sture, G.H., Halliwell, R.E., Thoday, K.L. et al (1995). Canine atopic disease; the prevalence of positive intradermal skin tests at two sites in the north and south of Great Britain. *Veterinary Immunology and Immunopathology* **44**, 293–308.

Vink, A.A., Strickland, F.M., Bucana, C., Cox, P.A., Roza, L. and Yarosh, D.B. (1996). Localization of DNA damage and its role in altered antigen–presenting cell function in ultraviolet-irradiated mice. *Journal of Experimental Medicine* **183**, 1491–1500.

Yager, J.A. and Wilcock, B.P. (1994). *Color Atlas and Text of Surgical Pathology of the Dog and Cat.* Wolfe Publishing, London.

Veterinarians and Responsible Pet Ownership

12

Caroline Jevring, Thomas E. Catanzaro

> *Do we understand the commitment a pet requires from us and are we returning to them the devotion we owe?*
>
> Marty Becker, DVM

Animal ownership is not a random event: acceptance or rejection of the relationship requires conscious effort and energy. As a result, pet-owners are often broadly divided into those who are 'responsible' and those who are not. Pets have moved from the backyard to the bedroom: more and more often, pets have family member status. The responsible pet-owner owns a pet that is very important in making them feel wanted and needed: in return, the owner cares diligently and, usually, lovingly for the pet.

Much is said and written about the importance of 'responsible pet ownership', but what exactly does it mean? The term 'responsible' must include a number of qualities:

- an appreciation of and delight in animals;
- understanding of the needs and behaviour of animals;
- involvement in and commitment to the human–animal bond;
- consideration of the value of human–animal relationships for the benefit of people and society;
- respect for life and quality of life.

An appreciation of and delight in animals

The joy that comes from owning a responsive, playful, and apparently loving companion is quite wonderful (Fig. 12.1). Your pet is always glad to see you whatever the rest of the world may feel! There is also the pleasure that comes from watching pets, at rest or play. Anyone who has owned a cat appreciates the beauty of their sinuous grace, laughs when they chase a ball, or feels calmed by the rasp of their purr.

Often this appreciation is extended to other animals too, such as watching lambs skipping in a field, cows contentedly chewing the cud, or a deer standing in a forest clearing. The pleasure given by these sights is felt at a deep level within the senses. There is a warm feeling of connection with Nature and natural things.

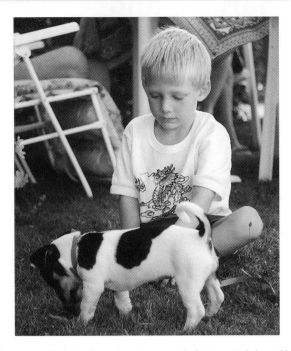

Fig. 12.1 The joy people derive from close contact with their pets is balanced by the veterinarian's responsibility to help them keep the pet in the best of health, for the pet's sake and for their own. © Ann F. Stonehouse.

Understanding of the needs and behaviour of animals

A veterinary behaviour specialist once shared the tale of two puppies, one of whom was dead before it was a year old. He showed slides of a cuddly, flop-eared Springer Spaniel and a squash-faced American Pit Bull Terrier and asked the audience to guess which one had died unnecessarily. Most chose the Pit Bull — but, in fact, that had grown to be a well-disciplined, well-behaved adult. It was the Springer Spaniel puppy who had been euthanased for behaviour problems. The cute growling the little pup would do when it settled on a sofa cushion was not so funny when the owner was bitten in the face trying to remove the young adult from 'its' place on the sofa. This puppy had never been taught the social behaviour that would have made it an enjoyable family member.

Understanding of the needs and behaviour of animals must include understanding of the needs and behaviour of the people who will own the animal, and how the two can fit together. The traumatic breakdown of the human–pet bond and elective euthanasias of young pets most frequently occurs because the two are not well matched.

Responsible pet ownership starts with selecting the right pet and then caring for it in such a way as to make it an enjoyable and rewarding companion. Creating an enjoyable and rewarding companion includes appropriate training and behavioural management. Often, the 'undesirable' behaviour that causes untimely death is actually normal for the animal, although it may be exaggerated by the situation into which the animal is forced. For example, it is normal for cats to sharpen their claws by scratching on hard surfaces, typically the bark of a tree. Increasingly, however, people keep cats permanently shut in their houses or flats, and the cats use and damage furniture with their actions. Forcing the cat into an unnatural situation creates 'undesirable' behaviour. In the United States, owners will declaw their cats as an alternative to euthanasia.

Similarly, dogs are social pack animals who do not like to be left on their own for prolonged periods of time. In many households, dogs are left on their own for most of the day which leads to boredom, loneliness and frustration and may result in destructive behaviour. Again, the 'undesirable' behaviour results from forcing the animal into an unnatural situation. The answer lies in selection of a more appropriate pet that better suits the owner's life-style, or a commitment to helping the pet express its energies more naturally. For example, in recognition of this need for social contact, some responsible owners take their dogs to 'play school' where they have the chance to meet other dogs, play and exercise.

Sexual management of pets is also an important part of creating an enjoyable and rewarding companion. Animals have innate needs and drives: a continually sexually frustrated male dog or cat may be aggressive to other animals and show undesirable behaviour towards humans. Owners must understand that for their pet to fit comfortably into *human* society these innate behaviours must be reduced, which is achieved through early neutering (see Chapter 8).

Involvement in and commitment to the human–animal bond

'A dog is for life' is the motto of organisations promoting responsible pet care such as the Delta Organisation in the United States. A pet is essentially dependent on its owner. A responsible owner makes a commitment to care for their pet when they choose to take stewardship of it, which includes catering to the physical and mental needs of the animal. This differs between breeds and species – a large dog, for example, may need several miles of exercise daily and strong behavioural management, whereas a long-haired cat needs daily grooming but could live its life indoors. These needs may change over the animal's lifetime, but the commitment to care cannot.

The veterinarian is the spokesperson for the health and welfare of the pet and is part of the family–pet bond (Fig. 12.2). Owners who are truly committed to the bond they have created with their pets regard regular contact with a trusted veterinarian as integral to their stewardship.

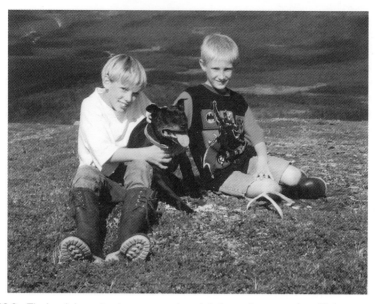

Fig. 12.2   The bond that exists between people and their pets is very precious. Veterinarians have a special role to nurture, honour and celebrate that bond.

Consideration of the value of human–animal relationships for the benefit of people and society

The importance and value of human–animal interactions have been copiously documented. Pets are good for human health; for example, studies show that people who own pets typically visit the doctor less often and use less medication. Pet-owners on average have lower cholesterol and lower blood pressure. They recover more quickly from illness and surgery, and they deal better with stressful situations. However, the *significance* of this information is not being exploited as it should be.

Only a few generations ago people were brought up in much closer contact with animals and Nature. This had many implications, from the calming effect of seeing animals quietly living their lives and following the natural flow of the seasons, to giving their owners a role and place in society. Most people's livelihoods and lives relied on animal power and selling animal products; for the upper classes, high-bred horses and dogs were symbols of status and wealth.

Now people grow up in an increasingly animal-free environment. Schools forbid 'small furries' because of the alarming increase in allergy amongst children. People elect not to have pets because they do not fit in with their hectic life-style. Elderly people are forced to give up their pets when they move into sheltered housing. The rich own Mercedes cars and Rolex watches. City-dwellers experience less and less contact with Nature and the natural cycles of life, and the incidence of stress and stress-related diseases is ever-increasing.

Encouraging caring ownership of an appropriate pet would be of vast benefit to individuals and society as a whole. Pets offer companionship, social contact with other owners, something to laugh at and with, a reason to exercise, and they create feelings of self-worth for their owners. No-one appreciates you as much as your pet does! Responsible owners know this and do their best to champion the pet in society.

Respect for life and quality of life

Caring owners believe that animals have a right to live and enjoy a reasonable quality of life. During health, this typically reflects the owner's quality of life. When the animal is severely ill or dying, the responsible pet-owner will, in conference with their veterinarian, make choices that reflect their concern and understanding for their pet's quality of life. These are based on such parameters as the ability of the animal to eat, groom, and defaecate and urinate in the appropriate place.

Responsibilities for costs

Pet insurance is also an important part of responsible pet ownership. For a relatively low annual sum, owners can be protected against unexpected costly treatment for injured or sick pets. This means that financial considerations are not the limiting factor in treatment and also enables veterinarians to perform more comprehensive diagnostic and treatment protocols if necessary.

Of course, ensuring that a pet always stays in good health means the self-risk costs never need be paid either. But healthcare is not free. Well thought through payment plans for pet-owners on annual wellness programmes ensure a commitment from the owner to regular clinic visits, and provide a predetermined source of income for the practice. Owners can choose different levels of wellness care and different levels of cost, and can choose to pay this annually or divided into monthly instalments.

What is an irresponsible pet-owner?

An *irresponsible* pet-owner is one who does not display some or all of the qualities described above. Lack of responsibility is recognised to be part of the inertia associated with the needless suffering and death of millions of unwanted and homeless animals every year.

An irresponsible pet-owner does not have an appreciation for and delight in animals and is often indifferent towards animals, seeing them as disposable items.

An irresponsible pet-owner does not include the veterinarian as part of the human–pet bond. One veterinary organisation affiliated to a major pet chainstore notes that over 50% of their clients have never seen a veterinarian or have not visited one in the last 18 months. Where are these owners getting the information and medical advice they need to care properly for their pet?

Irresponsible pet-owners create social conflict and stress: their animals pollute the environment, threaten the lives of people and other creatures, breed indiscriminately, spread diseases, cause road accidents, and so on. Poorly managed dogs and cats that run loose, soil property, and bark or yowl indiscriminately are bad ambassadors. In addition, people who keep so many animals that they are a nuisance for the whole community reinforce the stereotype that animal ownership is linked with misanthropy.

Irresponsible pet-owners may have a very confused attitude towards what constitutes respect for life and other living things.

> *On a holiday in Greece, my husband and I sat in a restaurant watching a large Greek family enjoy their meal. The family matriach had a small Chihuahua sitting on her knee that she hand-fed with scraps of meat from her own plate, and she frequently bestowed kisses and other signs of affection on her pet. Hanging from the back of her chair with a string tied tightly around its slowly desiccating body, was a large land snail. Its attempts to draw itself into the protection of its shell became weaker and weaker as dinner progressed. Appalled, we asked the proprietor of the restaurant what they were doing.*
>
> *'Oh, they just want its shell,' he replied airily. 'No problem.'*
>
> *We left.*

The dilemmas

Naturally, there are dilemmas. Who defines responsibility – owners or non-owners? Pet-owners are often remarkably uncritical about the problems caused by their pets. They also, not surprisingly, have more positive and emotional feelings for pets than do non-owners. Non-owners may regard animals as nuisances, or creatures to be feared. This feeling often stems from a mixture of old wives' tales (many people still fear cats because of their historical connection with witches and black forces), childhood experiences such as being bitten by a large dog, and the environment where the child grew up where, for example, one or both parents were afraid of animals, animals were not allowed in the house because of allergy, or the parents themselves had no interest in or understanding for animals.

As owners and non-owners are forced to co-exist, often very closely in the urban situation, it is important that both groups share an honest perception, thus making it possible to develop strategies that could meet the needs of both. Pets can be wonderful for many people and at least an accepted if not a welcomed part of the urban setting for most other people if they are maintained in a wholesome and responsible way.

Sadly, there is a notable lack of understanding by city planners, architects, school systems and legislators: despite the proven benefits of pet ownership, it is becoming more difficult to own pets in many cities around the world. Dogs are banned in many urban parks and places for open-air public bathing. Pet ownership is being compromised in the push for urban consolidation: smaller backyards discourage people from owning pets. More than 140 000 pets are taken to veterinarians or animal sanctuaries each year when their older owners move into new accommodation in the United Kingdom. Of these, 27% are subsequently put down, 40% are sent to or kept in rescue centres, and only 33% are actually rehomed. In some states in Australia, there is legislation limiting the number of pets people are permitted to own, and affecting the ownership of cats (Fig. 12.3).

The human–pet bond takes place within a cultural, social, and ecological environment that sets many of the parameters of normal, or, at least, acceptable behaviours and roles. These differ from country to country. In Britain, for example, acceptable dog ownership includes neutering the pet to prevent straying and unwanted puppies, but less than 10% of owners insure their pet against disease and injury. In Sweden, where there is a very low incidence of stray dogs and unwanted mating, neutering is not often performed but over 50% of dogs are insured. In the United States, all pets must be officially registered; this is not a requirement in most parts of Europe.

Attitudes towards pet ownership and what constitutes acceptable behaviours and roles within a society are extremely variable. In western society, pets may be the cherished companions of movie stars, politicians, and others requiring social approval (how much does American President Bill Clinton's cat 'Socks' affect his popularity rating? How much of Barbara Cartland's image is linked with her pampered Pekes?) – or they may be the cause of social conflict, and their owners are depicted as social hermits who have lost faith with their fellow humans (think of the people who 'rescue' animals and end up with hundreds packed into their council flat). Both extremes exist at the same time in the same society.

Cultural attitudes towards pets vary enormously. The relationship the nomadic-pastoralist Turkana of Northern Kenya have with their dogs, for example, could be described as a tolerant symbiosis. Their dogs are used as camp scavengers and watchdogs. They are rarely petted or caressed. They live much as the people do: if conditions are good in this semi-arid desert area and there has been plenty of rainfall, everyone is happy and well-fed; if conditions are bad, animals and people die. Compare this with a pampered Persian in a luxury apartment in up-town New York fed only on finest fresh steak. Or a pack mule in Morocco who, like his owner, works until he drops. Or a beloved overweight family Labrador in England.

Pets' quality of life largely reflects their owners' living standards. Even in western society, the quality of life for many owners falls well short of 'ideal'. For example, from lack of money and knowledge, they and their children eat nutritionally poor diets based on fried foods and fizzy drinks, and survive. Is it realistic to expect them to understand the need for and purchase nutritionally optimal (and often expensive) diets for their pets? Does this mean these owners are irresponsible?

Increasingly, in the never-ending search for novelty, exotic animals are becoming more popular. People keep as pets large spiders, scorpions and reptiles – creatures with whom it would appear to be more difficult to form an affectionate, loving relationship (identified as one of the key rewards in cat and dog ownership), and that in other cultures would be despised and feared. What is acceptable (responsible) owner behaviour in these situations?

Everyone who has a close relationship with a pet anthropomorphises the relation to some extent by, for example, interpreting actions and sounds into human behaviour and language, feeding their own food ('*Tibby loves haddock cooked in cream!*'), and so on. Mostly this is fairly harmless and is part of the enjoyment of pet ownership. Some people, however, blur the division between man and animal too much, making them into child substitutes or toys and insisting on giving them human desires and emotions ('*She must be allowed to breed naturally to be fulfilled!*'), even going so far as to dress them up and 'marry' them to each other in mock ceremonies.

'Quality of life' becomes a particularly delicate issue where euthanasia is involved. Hospice-style care is increasingly available in the United States for terminally ill companion animal patients and will, no doubt, spread soon to Europe. The concept is that the animal can be kept alive longer if it is pain-free and well nursed, but is this truly giving the pet life quality? Should life quality be defined from the owner's or the pet's viewpoint? In many European countries, cancer therapy for pets is still not regularly practised because 'they are only animals' and the treatment is being performed 'to satisfy selfish human needs'. Yet many pets have been able to live longer in apparent good health because of such treatment, which has been tremendously rewarding for their devoted owners. In some cases, the limiting factor to quality of life for pets is the ideas and prejudices of the veterinarian himself.

The veterinarian and responsible pet ownership

Far from being a luxury, pets are increasingly becoming a necessity. The therapeutic, emotional and social roles of dogs and cats is expanding. Reality shows that as family, neighbour, and community bonds diminish the family–pet–vet bond increases. Having 'someone' to care for gives meaning to life, a reason to get up in the morning, a reason to want to come home at night. Pets satisfy the need to be needed and loved, an emotion that runs deep in all of us, regardless of age, colour, sex or economic success.
Marty Becker

The practice of veterinary medicine involves people, animals, and the environment in which they live. The veterinarian makes decisions that affect the emotional, physical, social, economic, and political well-being of clients and others in the community. As an integral part of the family–pet–vet team, the veterinarian has, therefore, a major role in defining and helping owners achieve responsible pet ownership. In fact, one of the key roles for veterinarians is to help owners retain the correct perspective on what is truly best for their pet.

However, it is only in the last decade or so that veterinarians have begun really to take on this role – perhaps as a reflection of the rapid increase in numbers of women in the profession, perhaps because over three quarters of income in veterinary practices comes from treating companion animals, perhaps because the continued growth of factory farming methods forecasts an even greater reduction in the need for agriculture-based veterinary services, or perhaps because of a general humanistic enlightenment in veterinary colleges reflected by an increasingly secure place for companion animal studies.

The veterinarian must rely on people to present their pets for clinical care and so he or she becomes intimately and inescapably involved in issues that affect the emotional health of the pet-owner and their family. To deal effectively with clients' emotions and needs as they relate to the psychodynamics of pet ownership, the veterinarian must have a sound knowledge base and effective verbal and non-verbal skills, including the arts of asking questions, observing and listening. Much of the role of the veterinarian is as a teacher. Effective teaching is achieved through sensitive awareness of a pupil's needs and fulfilling the desire for knowledge. This is especially critical in the family–pet–veterinarian relationship where the benefactor of the knowledge is not the pupil – the pet-owner – but the pet.

Healthcare programmes are a way of teaching pet-owners to care better for their pets. They help owners create the right environment for wellness in a step-by-step fashion. To be successful, it is essential to have the understanding and cooperation of the pet-owner. Without this understanding and trust the owner will not allow the veterinarian to treat their animal and will not follow his recommendations. The pet-owner is under the influence of many other persuasive voices (see Box 12.1). Successful wellness healthcare depends on the veterinarian's ability to communicate clearly and empathetically with the owner.

The need for change

It was not long ago that the human–pet bond was seen as misplaced sentimentality, so it is not surprising that many veterinarians are still resistant to practising wellness

---

Box 12.1 *Factors influencing clients*

- Friends, neighbours
- Breeders:
  A middle-aged lady with a 14-year-old poodle visited our surgery for the first time recently. The poodle had a massive mammary tumour that was ruptured and stinking. 'I'm afraid there's not much I can do here,' I explained gently. 'Why didn't you come to us earlier?'
  'Oh, I've been in constant touch with my breeder,' she replied. 'She advised me that breast tumours in dogs are inoperable – that it's worthless even trying at the early stages, they always grow back.'

- Previous experiences
- Advertising by producers of petcare products
- Pet shops
- Relationship with pet
- Their own health and living standards

healthcare in companion animal practice. There are a number of features of the way veterinary medicine is taught and practised that need to be changed to make wellness healthcare become truly active:

- *Student selection and training:* many veterinary students have not been exposed whilst they were growing up, or when seeing practice, to healthcare in action for their own or others' pets; most companion animal practices still practise reactive medicine.

- Wellness programmes will not work unless they take place in *the right environment*. Companion animal veterinarians must learn to present their practices as places to bring healthy animals not simply treat sick ones.

  An elderly lady visited our practice recently with her new Cavalier King Charles puppy for vaccination. As I walked into the reception area he greeted me ecstatically, his whole body wagging and his eyes bright with the excitement of making a new friend.

  'Of course, he shouldn't really be here,' said the lady apologetically. 'He's not sick at all – he's only come for his vaccinations.'

- *Better communication with clients:* veterinarians are not taught to go out to clients proactively and talk about disease prevention and wellness in companion animals. They learn how to treat sickness, and expect their clients to know when to come to them to seek help. This approach is outdated and is increasingly not what clients want. If veterinarians do not change their attitude promptly, they will lose out to breeders, pet-shops, and other knowledgeable people and organisations who apparently provide the information pet-owners seek.

- *Learn to teach clients about better pet care.* This is a long-term activity requiring a high level of commitment. It takes time and energy. A teacher-veterinarian should not 'talk and tell' to his clients but gently persuade them to 'buy' his ideas. The veterinarian is 'selling' a product that is very familiar to him: it is obvious to him what all the advantages are. But that often blinds veterinarians to what their clients are interested in. For example, daily toothbrushing is accepted as being the most effective way of controlling dental plaque in dogs and cats, but how many veterinarians brush their own pet's teeth on a daily basis? How can the veterinarian then recommend this as the best way to manage plaque if he himself does not have the time, energy, ability, desire, etc.

Box 12.2 *Proactive client teaching methods*

- Talk to your clients at every opportunity
- Use handouts
- Use videos
- Send newsletters
- Send mail reminders for preventive healthcare actions, e.g. vaccinations
- Demonstrate using models, e.g. of healthy and diseased teeth and gums
- Supply the healthcare products you recommend, e.g. optimum quality foods, parasite control products

---

to perform this on his own pet? Similarly, how can he recommend X brand of pet food as being the best for his clients' pets if he does not feed it to his own pet?

- *Learn to listen to clients:* veterinarians are typically taught to 'fix problems'. Pet-owners have a very different viewpoint about animal care from the veterinarian. Their pets are primarily for pleasure: getting people to care for their pets is not about making them feel guilty. What is important is that the veterinarian *listens* to the client and adapts his knowledge to best suit the client's and the pet's needs.

    An example of this is when helping an owner to diet an overweight dog. You will gain far better compliance from the owner if you allow him or her to continue giving the beloved pet a good-night treat – perhaps a portion of the diet food, or some sort of low calorie snack – than if you completely forbid this important interaction.

- *Make a commitment to work constant with wellness healthcare.* There is enough evidence and scientific knowledge to prove that prevention is better than cure. By talking about wellness at every opportunity, packaging wellness into clearly labelled groups of services, demonstrating care (tooth-brushing techniques, how to give worm medicine, simple behavioural commands such as 'Sit!' and 'Lie!'), making sure clients never leave the clinic without at least some information about better wellness care for their pets, and going out to clients with mailed information and treatment reminders, the veterinarian is able to guide his clients effectively towards better pet care.

The human–animal bond and ethics

Let us be aware that grief for pet animals is more than just an overflow for draining emotion. It is also a springboard for awakening our moral concern for the millions of creatures whose lives are wasted and twisted in our hands, and yet for whom no tears are shed.
Rollin, 1984

The human–animal bond is complex: on the one hand man can love a companion animal like a child, on the other he can condone the brutal daily slaughter of creatures reared for their meat. Companion animals have a moral status, possess intrinsic value, and are legitimate objects of moral concern and attention towards whom our actions must be judged in terms of right and wrong. This is something we feel intuitively, and which is easily felt and expressed emotionally (as when we grieve for pets). However, it is very difficult to give a philosophical and rational articulation to this sense of animal value without sliding into terms perceived by many as sloppy sentimentality.

Historically various reasons have been given for cruelty to animals, ranging from the religious one that animals have no soul, to the Cartesian assertion that animals are merely machines and can therefore feel no pain. Depersonalisation appears to be an important component in the mistreatment of animals, as in giving laboratory animals numbers rather than names.

Recently, a new level of responsibility has started to emerge amongst people and societies: stewardship. Stewardship entails constant monitoring of every human interaction in any biological system, including natural ecosystems, ranging from such things as oceans and wilderness habitats to man-made systems and the soil of our farmlands, from the genetics and metabolism of high-yield dairy cattle to the gait and temperament of a German Shepherd. The physical and psychological degeneration and emotional problems of companion animals, for example, necessitate concerted stewardship from veterinarians, pet-owners and breeders.

Veterinarians are amongst that group of people who are concerned about the plight of animals and seek to narrow the ethical gulf that separates members of our own species from members of other species in our conventional morality. The average person who acquires a cat or dog is often infused with outrageously false information ranging from 'Dogs and cats are natural enemies and can't live together' to 'The way to house-train a dog is to hit it when it defaecates or rub its nose in the excrement'. As a result, most violations against pet animals' rights occur through ignorance not deliberate cruelty. It is the job of veterinarians to teach owners about the normal needs and behaviours of their pets, and how best to care for them.

Shortly after moving to Sweden, my oldest son, then aged seven, was asked during his English lessons about opposites. Up? – down. Left? – right. Black? – white. Cat? Cat?

He was absolutely stumped, and eventually came home furiously angry with his teacher who had insisted that the opposite of cat was dog. 'But we've always had cats and dogs living happily together,' he said. 'They're not opposites – they're friends!'

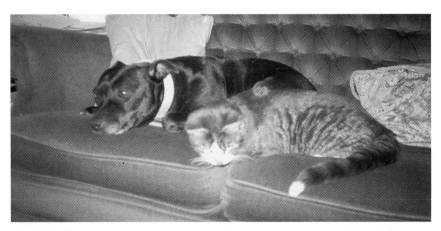

Fig. 12.3 Many people keep more than one pet. The veterinarian has a key role in advising on responsible pet ownership.

The future: bond-centred practices

The term 'bond-centred practice' was developed by Laurel Lagoni, Carolyn Butler and Susanne Hetts within the context of their clinical work in the Support for People and Pets Programme at Colorado State University. In a bond-centred practice, veterinary care is focused where the medical needs of animals and the emotional needs of their human owners coincide. This conjunction or point of attachment is referred to as the human–animal bond. In a bond-centred practice the unique significance of each human–animal relationship is assessed and respectfully acknowledged, and the needs of the animal patients and human owners are simultaneously addressed. This is accomplished by providing high quality medical-based and support-based services, extending veterinary care beyond the medical treatment of companion animals.

In April 1998, the first meeting of a new veterinary organisation was held. VetOne has two simple objectives:

1   to increase the number of bonded pet-owners, that is to increase the number of responsible companion animal owners who utilise veterinary services at a preferred level (pets-as-children);
2   to increase the number of veterinarians providing 'bond-centred' service.

The founder, Dr Marty Becker, set down the mission of this meeting as:
To shine an illuminating energising light on this global phenomenon called the family–pet–veterinary bond and look at what our unique opportunities and responsibilities are as related to 'the bond'. As pets are increasingly being treated as family members, what can we do to celebrate and protect this powerful affection connection in a way that optimises the health, happiness and longevity of pets and people, and in a manner that will benefit all stakeholders?

Some final thoughts

Veterinarians are integral to the family–pet bond. Let's go into the twenty-first century with a firm commitment to not only fix sick animals but also help people really cherish their animals! Let's make a commitment to teaching responsible pet ownership! Let's make a commitment to pet healthcare! Let's make a commitment to truly celebrate the family–pet–veterinarian bond!

References and further reading

Anchor Trust report quoted in *Veterinary Record*, May 23rd, 1998.

Australian Companion Animal Council (1995). *The Power of Pets*. September 1995, P.O. Box 371, Artarman, New South Wales, 2064.

Braun, E. (1984) The human–animal bond revisited. In: Kay, W.J. et al (eds) *Pet Loss and Human Bereavement*. Iowa State Press, De Moines, Iowa, pp 111–118.

Bustad, L. and Hines, L. (1981) A curriculum to promote greater understanding of the human–companion animal bond. In: Fogle, B. (ed) *Interrelations between People and Pets*. Charles C. Thomas, Springfield, Illinois, pp 241–267.

Catanzaro, T.E. (1992). Why are there too many euthanasias? *Latham Letter* **XIII**(4), 1,7,8.

Catanzaro, T.E. (1998) *Building the Successful Veterinary Practice: Innovation & Creativity* (Vol. 3). Iowa State University Press, Ames, Iowa.

Fox, M. (1981) Relationships between the human and non-human animals. In: Fogle, B. (ed) *Interrelations between People and Pets*. Charles C. Thomas, Springfield, Illinois, pp 23–40.

Lagoni, L., Butler, C. and Hetts, S. (1994). *The Human–Animal Bond and Grief*. W.B. Saunders, London.

Rollin, B.E. (1983). Morality and the human–animal bond. In: Katcher, A.H. and Beck, A.M. (eds) *New Perspectives on our Lives with Companion Animals*. University of Pennsylvania Press, Philadelphia, pp 500–510.

Appendix I
Working with Clients

Client information sheets

The purpose of these handouts is to give clear, specific instructions or information in simple terms about disease prevention and management or pet healthcare. Such handouts:

- give the owner a better understanding of particular health problems;
- give the owner advice on home care/management;
- give answers to common questions;
- inform owners of the benefits of new or existing services/products in the practice to the benefit of themselves and their pets.

Information sheets can be personalised with the client's and the pet's name and with information specific to their particular problem (if the practice has a computer).

Some helpful tips

- Check spelling and grammar if you write your own handouts. Misspellings and bad grammar detract from a professional appearance. There is no excuse for poor layout with the simple-to-use desk-top publishing systems now available.
- If you use pre-printed information from, for example, vaccine companies, make sure you have read the information yourself and that it agrees with practice policy. For example, one brochure on general pet care that a practice was interested in using recommended neutering dogs (both males and females) before six months of age, which was not acceptable in that practice.
- Fewer than 15% of clients will read a handout if it is just taken from a rack. Make sure you actively put it in the client's hands with the words, 'Read this, it's important and please feel free to ask us any questions you may have'. This will increase the reading rate to nearer 85%.
- Include appropriate leaflets in an information pack. For example, a kitten pack could include leaflets on nutrition, vaccination, worming, neutering, pet insurance, and the facilities in the practice.
- Post information to clients rather than lose time trying to explain things on the phone.

Videos

There are an increasing number of high quality educational videos available. These are produced by pet product manufacturers and can be invaluable teaching aids for clients. Ideally, the client should be able to look at the videos in a quiet, undisturbed location and then have the opportunity to ask questions and discuss the contents with an informed staff member. In some cases, owners may be able to borrow videos to study at home.

Video teaching should be used selectively: recent studies have indicated that clients do not always like video as they feel it cuts them off from human contact.

Practices can also sell information videos. They can provide a useful supplement to educational books. One feline practice I visited sold videos for home-viewing – for the cats, not the owners! They sold like hotcakes to enchanted owners!

Newsletters

A short, well-written newsletter sent out to clients several times a year is an ideal way of updating and informing clients about healthcare activities. Newsletters should not be long, both because they take more time to write and because length is not an index of readability.

The biggest problem with newsletters is often that, in the beginning, the practice is very enthusiastic and has great ambitions for frequently sending out a fancy newsletter. After a time, everyone runs out of steam and the whole project fizzles out.

Some tips in writing a good newsletter are:
- Don't send it out more often than three or four times a year.
- Keep it short and to the point (we send a double-sided A4 newsletter).
- Don't make articles too long or technical.
- Include some friendly personal information about the practice and its members.
- Keep costs down by producing a quality product using a desk-top publishing system.
- Make sure the practice name, logo, address, telephone number and opening times are clearly displayed.
- Use colour, for example coloured paper or coloured envelopes, to attract attention.

Internet websites

The latest way of contacting and informing clients is via Internet websites. Some very lively and exciting examples of these exist, even including real-time contact with hospitalised or boarded pets. Websites offer a personalised, attractive, and easily updated method of:

- informing clients about practice services;
- giving clients examples of real-case situations;
- answering common questions about routine care such as vaccinations, worming, bathing, and so on;
- enabling clients to have an input in the care of their pet when travelling or away from a telephone.

On the downside, websites are expensive to set up, and it is not yet clear how many clients actively visit the sites.

Additional information on forms, newsletters, client-bonding and internal promotion can be found in the new thee Volume series – *Building the Successful Veterinary Practice: Leadership Tools (Vol. 1); Programs & Procedures (Vol. 2); Innovation & Creativity (Vol. 3)* – by Thomas E. Catanzaro, DVM, MHA, FACHE, (1998) Iwoa State University Press, Ames, Iwoa, USA.

Recommended Further Reading for Clients

Appleby, D. *How to have a happy puppy.* Available from APBC, PO Box 46, Worcester, WR8 9YS, England.

Appleby, D. *How to have a contented cat.* Available from APBC, PO Box 46, Worcester, WR8 9YS, England.

Appleby, D. *Ain't Misbehavin' Broadcast Books.* 4, Cotham Vale, Bristol, BS6 6HR, England.

Bailey, G. (1995) *Perfect Puppy.* Hamlyn, Michelin House, 81, Fulham Road, London, SW3 6RB, England.

Bessant, C. and Viner, V. *The Ultrafit Older Cat.* Smith Gryphon Limited, Swallow House, 11-21 Northdown Street, London, N1 9BN, England.

Dunbar, I. (1991) *Doctor Dunbar's Good Little Dog Book.* James and Kenneth Publishers, 2140 Shattuck Avenue, #2406 Berkley, California 94704, USA.

Dunbar, I. (1996) *How to teach a new dog old tricks.* James and Kenneth Publishers, 2140 Shattuck Avenue, #2406 Berkley, California 94704, USA.

Edney, A. (1992) *Complete Cat Care Manual.* RSPCA, Published by Doring Kindersley Limited, 9 Henrietta Street, London WC2E 8PS, England.

Edney, A. (1992) *Complete Dog Care Manual.* RSPCA, Published by Doring Kindersley Limited, 9 Henrietta Street, London WC2E 8PS, England.

Evans, M. (1996) *The Complete Guide to Kitten Care,* Mitchell Beazley. Michelin House, 81, Fulham Road, London, SW3 6RB, England.

Evans, M. (1996) *The Complete Guide to Puppy Care.* Mitchell Beazley, Michelin House, 81, Fulham Road, London, SW3 6RB, England.

Fisher, J. (1993) *Why Does My Dog...?* Souvenir Press Ltd, 43 Great Russell Street, London, WC1B 3PA, England.

Heath, S. (1995) *Why Does My Cat...?* Souvenir Press Ltd, 43 Great Russell Street, London, WC1B 3PA, England.

Neville, P. Bessant, C. and Viner, V. *How to give your dog a longer and healthier life.* Available from APBC, PO Box 46, Worcester, WR8 9YS, England.

Neville, P. (1995) *Perfect Kitten,* Hamlyn, Michelin House, 81, Fulham Road, London, SW3 6RB, England.

Patmore, K. (1991) *So your children want a dog.* Popular Dogs, 20 Vauxhall Bridge Road, London, SW1V 2SA, England.

Index

Page numbers in italics refer to figures and tables